What the Bleep $#@! Can I Eat?

Are you having digestive issues? Do you have food allergies? Have you been diagnosed with Celiac disease? Do you have high blood sugar or cholesterol? Overweight? Confused about what you should eat?

Allergen-Free

Gluten-Free

Low Glycemic

High Fiber

Antioxidant-Rich

Omega 3 Balanced

Authored by Dr. Debra Anastasio, Naturopathic Doctor, who along with her two children, have Celiac disease and food allergies. Dr. Anastasio provides professional advice and practical suggestions for how to tackle the issue of what to eat both in your home and in restaurants. An invaluable guide to getting healthy and being happy in the process!

What the Bleep $#@! Can I Eat?

A Family Guide for Healthy Eating

Published by Jinny Hill Press

Printed by Lulu Enterprises, Inc.

www.lulu.com

ISBN 978-0-557-35413-9

This book is dedicated to all of my patients, family and friends. Eat well, feel well, and be well! I wish you the best health and happiness possible.

Contents

Recipe List

What the Bleep $#@! Can I Eat?

Fresh Berry Pie with Nut Crust	82
Oat Protein Bars	97
Whole grain pilaf	97
Loaded Sweet Potato	98
Cold Tabouleh Salad	105
Three Bean Salad	106
Black Eyed Pea Salad	106
Shredded Slaw	106
Black Bean Chutney	106
Turkey Chili	107
Antioxidant Smoothie	114
Fruit & Nut Truffles	115
Breakfast Hash	115
Roasted Herbed Sweet Potatoes	115
Chicken/Tofu Curry	116
Antioxidant All-Purpose Marinade	116
Antioxidant All-Purpose Salad Vinaigrette	116

What the Bleep $#@! Can I Eat?

What the Bleep $#@! Can I Eat?

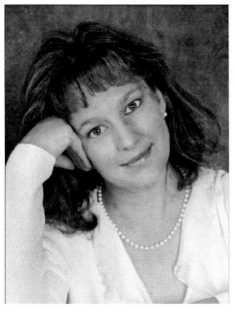

Dr. Debra Anastasio, is the founder and clinical director of the New England Naturopathic Center in Cheshire, CT. Dr. Anastasio is also the past President of the Connecticut Naturopathic Physicians Association and past professor at the University of Bridgeport, College of Naturopathic Medicine. She is also a preceptor for Naturopathic medical students in her office and a professional member of the American Association of Naturopathic Physicians.

Dr. Anastasio is a natural health author for Livestrong.com and local health magazines. She also presents seminars, is a guest lecturer for universities and organizations, and creates retreats for the public and patients to attend.

Dr. Debra writes a "Monday Morning Blahg", "Tuesday Tweet of the Week", has an internet radio show "Thank Goodness I'm Healthy" and has health discussions on Facebook. Dr. Anastasio also has a supplement line called "Metamorphosis Products that is referenced in the book as an example of quality supplements."

www.drdebraanastasio.com

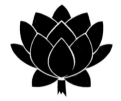

Introduction: Are you ready to eat healthy?

Everyone needs to improve their diet, but what happens when you have to? Nobody likes having to give up their favorite foods if they're on the list of no-no's! After dishing out the news to patients that they can't eat their favorite foods, they often reply "What the $#@! Can I Eat?" This book is a bridge from the unhealthy eating habits of typical Americans to a healthier diet with mass appeal. It is not a macrobiotic, vegetarian, raw food book, strictly health food diet because most people are not ready for that extreme of a change all at once. This is a practical approach for most people to dramatically improve their health by incorporating simple healthy foods in their diet.

I have written one too many meal plans, have looked endlessly for the right books to recommend that all have their shortcomings, and have answered endless calls from patients at the grocery store asking about a certain food or ingredient that finally made me cry "Uncle!" This book is long overdue and sorely needed by my patients, and me, and hopefully for the rest of you!

What the Bleep $#@! Can I Eat?

What the Bleep $#@! Can I Eat? delivers information and suggestions for eating allergy-free, gluten-free, low glycemic, high fiber, antioxidant-rich, and omega-3 balanced meals. There is a section dedicated to each topic, a comprehensive meal planning guide, and tips for eating out so you can understand how to apply the principles of healthy eating no matter where you go!

I understand that drastically changing your diet can be scary and confusing, but it won't be any more, that is if you listen to me ☺! I can't tell you how many times patients [and family] ignore what I tell them, only to hear them at some future time and place tell me how they just discovered on Dr. Oz, or in Prevention Magazine about "X, Y or Z" food to improve their health. For example, "Did you know that taking apple cider vinegar can get rid of digestive problems?" I'm sure the look of surprise on my face is misinterpreted as excitement at such a discovery. Do I care how you learn it or accept it? No. I just want you to finally get it and do it! Proper nutrition is the number one medicine of choice for the treatment and prevention of the majority of diseases that affect people today, yet so few people are willingly changing before there is a serious problem to face.

Perhaps eating healthier is more challenging because of busy schedules, but it is also difficult because there is very little support in our society to eat right. The message being sent to you is the exact opposite of healthy: eat fast, look for huge portions, and treat yourself because you 'deserve it.' Guilty pleasures will not make you feel better . . . ever! Instead, why not make sure you enjoy life. You won't be thinking you deserved to get cancer or a heart attack when it happens, but your diet would be partly to blame.

It's like when a smoker gets diagnosed with lung cancer, is there any real great surprise? When Diabetics eat sugar, bread, and pasta all the time, is it any surprise they lose their eyesight or their limbs? We offer a sympathetic, 'it's too bad this happened' attitude hoping they'll change. This may sound harsh, but this is what I see and hear in my office on a regular basis. I know you are all in control of your destiny for so many illnesses that I want all this craziness to stop! You need to be as healthy as you can be without falsely relying on medicines that you think are going to save you, because in the end, they probably won't if you keep eating unhealthy.

So, let me just say what this book is *not*. It is *not* truly a cookbook with recipe after recipe. Instead, it is a journey into *how* to eat healthy, and *why* to eat healthy, and a kick in the pants to get started eating healthy! You can't just sit around whining about your health problems, or sit idle feeling defeated with your latest diagnosis or new prescription. If you feel bad, you need to accept that you alone have the power to make a positive change in your life. The place to start is with what you eat. Period. When you eat better, you will feel better, and maybe you can get off the couch and do some exercises too!

Think about it this way, when you drive your car and the fuel warning light comes on, you instinctively know how far you can push it before you'll be stranded on the roadside calling for assistance. And for the times when you miscalculated and curse your way to a filling station by foot, did you learn your lesson or did it happen again? I can personally tell you this recently happened to me with great astonishment. I was moving so fast, with so many commitments, that I lost my instinct to fill up with gas in a reasonable time frame. It made me stop and think about how this represented what was happening in the rest of my life with my eating, with my sleep, with my downtime, with everything . . . I was running on empty! I responded by taking the long overdue vacation to put me back on firm footing, at least for the moment. This is something we have to keep working at, and when life gets busy, it gets harder. But that doesn't mean it's impossible to do!

Think of "What the Bleep $#@! Can I Eat?" as your food and eating guidebook. I want to help you get rid of the fear, resistance, confusion and upset of having to make a major diet change to improve your health. Most chronic diseases can be halted or even reverted by improving what you eat while avoiding toxic and expensive medicines. Don't you want this for yourself or your family? I can honestly tell you this is what I want for all of you! At least know what's possible and then decide for yourself how much you are willing to step in and get healthy. In these pages, I will give you the tools to succeed in your efforts while establishing a diet that not only solves one but many chronic health problems related to poor eating.

In case you didn't already see all the fanfare, the US Department of Agriculture has just released their new food guidelines for 2010! They apparently just figured out it is important to read labels for too much added salt, that Americans do not eat enough potassium-rich foods, and that trans-fats are to be avoided at all costs. Oh, and we're eating too many foods with nasty food additives that may actually be bad for us! Give me a break! My entire profession has known and taught this to patients for years!

Naturopathic doctors have been using parsley and dandelion leaf [loaded with potassium] to control blood pressure from too much sodium and not enough potassium in the diet. These same foods also help diabetics to control insulin and blood sugar. I guess we've come out of the dark ages thanks to the USDA! Jeez, I just can't wait for what they discover over the next five years for the next revision to save our sorry behinds![i]

What the Bleep $#@! Can I Eat?

Too bad they didn't emphasize that fiber from natural food sources prevents a multitude of diseases such as cancer, diabetes, high cholesterol, hormones imbalances that lead to reproductive cancer, gallbladder disease, bowel disease and more. It's a shame they don't tell people that organic foods are healthier and certain spices posses antioxidant power to protect and repair DNA damage of vital tissues, can prevent cancer, treat inflammation, repair damage, and offsetting the onslaught of environmental pollutants, such as food based pesticides! No, instead they are stuck in the same groove of sodium and fat [cholesterol] being bad, bad, bad and that avoiding them will somehow save you from certain death if you avoid them. Really? You be the judge when you read these pages!

You're about to learn what the food industry is doing to food that erodes your health and contributes to disease, and you're not going to like it! You're also not going to like it when I teach you about how organic really *is* better for you while the media and food industry would like you to think otherwise. For those of you 'going green' if you think that you're saving the environment with your hybrid cars or recycling efforts and you continue to use pesticide-laden foods, you have another thing to learn about the environment! You'll also learn about how there are no shortcuts to good health. Eat crap . . . feel like crap . . . end up dying of crap! No medicine is going to save you from all that crap you eat, so don't eat it!

Guess what, the "One Size Fits All Diet" in Chapter 9 accomplishes health [without the prompting of the U.S.D.A.] because I am teaching you to rely on *real foods* to live! Isn't that what you really want? To live a long, healthy life, or do you secretly have some death wish? We can only trust the food that nature [God and Mother Nature to be specific] provides. Stop cutting coupons or reading food ads and just focus on eating *real food* as the basis for every meal and snack with a minimal amount of prepared foods of the highest quality available!

You can find some healthy food at the regular grocer but I am challenging you to broaden your horizons. A trip to the health food store is not out of the question. Traversing the aisles of health food can feel like traveling to a foreign country. You won't recognize the packaging, the store smells like herbs, and things aren't as bright and shiny like you're used to, so it's a little less entertaining for those with short attention spans. It will probably be frustrating to eat healthy if all you rely on is shopping at the regular grocery store, and even more difficult at buyer's warehouses. Once you read *What the Bleep $#@! Can I Eat?,* you will have the tools to survive a trip to the health food store, the grocery store, and restaurants and get the healthy foods you need to succeed.

I can personally empathize with all of my patients when I prescribe diet changes for them. I recognize that most people are pretty happy eating the way that they do even when they know it is not good for them. There is a love affair with the taste buds getting what they want! Over the past few years both my children and I have been diagnosed with both food allergies and Celiac disease forcing us to make drastic changes in our diet. It doesn't matter what our taste buds might want, those foods make us sick and we can't have them. Sometimes I think that makes it easier because the foods are not even an option. I can tell you this, there are days that I wish I had a shortcut for a meal in 5 minutes from a drive-through, but that isn't an option for me, or my children, and it's not an option for you if you are suffering from any ill health.

Personal experience with a restricted food diet, combined with my clinical expertise treating patients that need dietary prescriptions, has become the foundation for making these recommendations because they are tried and true. This isn't based just on some theory or study, or even our wonderful U.S.D.A., these are broad reaching, practical ways to succeed at getting healthier through better eating. I can't be there to do it for you, so you have to learn to do this yourself!

I have purposefully avoided counting calories and grams of fats or carbohydrates for individual foods or meals. If you want to lose weight then adopt the O.S.F.A. diet and start exercising as your first two measures. I want you to develop a healthy relationship with food and trust what nature provides is what is good for you, while understanding that manufactured foods are a steep slope to ill health. Apples don't come with labels on them, and that is the point I want you to understand. Nature gets it right, what we do to the food in processing makes it all wrong. There is no magic diet to cure what ails you in one week or even one month. Adopting a healthy diet for the majority of the time over the span of months and years is what will make a difference in the end. When you adopt a healthy diet with consistency, your tissue will change for the better over time. This is what really works.

Is there room for treats and cheats? It depends on the person. Many people have addictive personalities, have struggled with food issues already, or lose control if they give themselves even a little of something they love that isn't good for them. You have to know yourself well enough to decide if a little wavering on the menu can be tolerated or not. Sweet and salty are addictive flavors and can trigger the nervous system to want more, and more, and more! MSG in foods helps this become a reality even more by making you eat far more than you would if the food did not contain MSG. Allergens have their own restrictions that will hold you back from cheating because the consequences are usually uncomfortable and sometimes deadly. Having Celiac, being on a gluten-free diet is an all or nothing experience, it leaves no room for cheating. For the rest of you, it takes willpower some of the time, support some of the time, and good planning most all of the time.

I know you can do this! Think of this book [me ☺] as your tour guide to healthy eating. You will stock your kitchens, plan meals and cook healthier than ever before. In the end, you will have a good idea of what to do, and what not to do, to save yourself from a multitude of diseases. Let your taste buds adjust to the change, it does get better with time! God Bless you all and I wish you great success in your eating endeavors.

--Dr. Anastasio

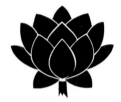

Chapter 1:
Optimizing Digestion

First, we need to make sure that your digestive system is fully up and running. If you are not digesting food properly, you will not benefit from all the nutrients your food can provide. Poor digestion can cause gas, bloating, constipation, diarrhea, bad breath, high cholesterol, hormone imbalances, food allergies, malnutrition or possibly inflammation that contributes to bowel disease or cancer. Some people are excessively hungry because they are not digesting properly and their cells are starving for nutrients. Take the time to follow these steps to optimize digestion before adopting your new way of eating. These measures alone can help you begin to feel better. This makes for a much more pleasurable and successful experience!

1. ONLY DRINK LIQUIDS BETWEEN MEALS

Water, mineral water, herbal tea, decaffeinated tea and decaffeinated coffee are the best liquid choices of all. These liquids hydrate your tissue, help produce secretions in your digestive tract, don't contain harmful chemicals, and help you make enough saliva. If you are well hydrated, there should be plenty of saliva present while you eat to help swallow your food.

At restaurants you are provided a large glass of ice water at the beginning of a meal. All that water mixes with your stomach acid and dilutes it to the point of not allowing the acid to break down the food. Instead of digesting, you begin fermenting which leads to gas, bloating, irritated gut lining, elevated blood sugar, weight gain, and problems with elimination.

Poor digestion and an irritated gut can lead to leaky gut that contributes to food allergies by allowing undigested proteins to reach your immune system. Your stomach acid is also responsible for triggering digestive juices from the pancreas and gall bladder. If this signal is drowned out by water, then your bile doesn't flow and cholesterol accumulates in the liver and raises cholesterol in the blood.

WHAT TO DO: Drink approximately 32-64 ounces of fluid throughout the day *between your meals* to optimize hydration and digestion.

2. SIT AND EAT CALMLY

Your nervous system is in charge of your digestion. If you are all excited, irritated, agitated, angry, or rushed, then the fight-or-flight part of your nervous system is in charge. Excitement of this nature prevents digestive juices from flowing freely and can lead to poor appetite, dry mouth, feeling too full on little food, and cravings for simple carbohydrates that are easy to digest quickly as opposed to complicated food proteins and whole grains that require digestive strength. Working while eating or picking on food while you feed the family keeps you in the stress mode and prevents proper digestion. In other words, stress makes you eat junk and feel like junk!

When you sit, say grace, and eat in an orderly manner, the nervous system calms down and signals to the gut that it is ready for food. Saliva and digestive juices flow easily to receive the food and break it down so you receive the nutrients it has to provide. You will be more equipped to handle a variety of proteins, fats, carbohydrates and fibers that are part of a healthy diet. Sitting actually helps the nervous system calm down and receive the meal in a more natural manner.

WHAT TO DO: Sit at a table with a clean, nice table setting to eat your meal. Say a prayer of grace or something nice and gracious about the food you are about to eat, or at the very least, thank the cook even if it was you!

3.   EAT NO MORE OFTEN THAN EVERY THREE HOURS and NO LESS THAN THREE REGULAR MEALS A DAY

For those who are hypoglycemic, eating every three hours becomes a way of life. Some people like to graze all day long on a variety of finger foods or grab-n-go foods because they are too busy or stressed to slow down and eat a real meal. And yet other people seem to barely eat at all throughout the day and start gorging on food when the sun starts to go down.

Your body is designed to receive food upon waking, at high noon and at dusk. These signals come from hormones that are part of your day-night regulation. If we honor the natural order of digestion, there would be no sleeping-in with late breakfasts or staying up late and eating into midnight hours. Erratic eating contributes to poor digestion, elevated blood sugar, weight gain, high cholesterol, and fatigue. The more tired you are, the more you will crave simple carbohydrates and not want healthy wholesome foods.

WHAT TO DO: Eat breakfast within 30 minutes of waking and before 8 a.m., eat lunch around noon, eat dinner before 7 p.m., and a light snack in the evening if needed. Make sure you are upright for 1 ½-2 hours after your last meal/snack so that digestion is completed before you lay down in bed.

4. STIMULATE DIGESTIVE JUICES

The most natural way to stimulate digestion is to use aromatic herbs and spices while cooking to begin the process of wanting the food. Use items from the onion/garlic family, savory herbs such as oregano, thyme, rosemary and basil, or spicy herbs such as chili pepper, ginger, or cinnamon.

Next is to have food that is pleasing to the eye and not just a pile of mush in a bowl. A variety of color on the plate is more pleasing than everything being tan or brown. Keep on hand some parsley or cilantro for garnishing and eating with the meal.

A pleasant eating environment is also recommended which means a kitchen or dining area that is free of clutter, that is clean [using only natural products instead of harsh chemicals], and nice tableware [as opposed to eating out of the pan or off of paper plates]. All too often people use their kitchen counters for piles of mail [bills] and then all you can think about is finances when you are eating. Another thing is that too many appliances or knick-knacks on the counters contribute to a crowded, stressful feeling in the kitchen. Keep the whole area free from anything that does not need to be out and put your papers at a desk or a separate room to be organized.

Using certain foods at the beginning of the meal will also stimulate digestion. Lemon in a small amount of water can be used at the beginning of a meal to help empty the stomach contents from the previous meal. Bitter greens such as dandelion, arugala, chickory, and endive can be eaten with lemon juice and olive oil at the beginning of the meal to stimulate stomach acid and bile flow. Organic apple cider vinegar [liquid not capsules] can be taken right before the meal to stimulate proper digestion. Use just one tablespoon by itself or in an ounce of water.

WHAT TO DO: De-clutter and clean the kitchen counters and dining table, use aromatic herbs in cooking, eat on nice plates, and use a digestive stimulant before the meal.

5. DIGESTIVE SUPPLEMENT AIDS

Digestive supplement aids mainly includes acids (glutamine and betaine), bitters, lecithin, enzymes, probiotics, and fibers and can be incredibly helpful for troubled digestive systems. For those of you on medications that reduce stomach acid, you need to consult a health practitioner about how to restart your digestive tract possibly with the help of digestive supplements.

Digestive Acids are necessary to digest your food, help your digestive organs function properly, and for absorption of vitamins, fats, and amino acids. Apple cider vinegar contains acetic acid and has long been used as a digestive aid in folk medicine and has made a comeback in recent years despite the fact that NIH or the USDA hasn't sanctioned its benefits. Lemon juice contains citric acid and has long been recommended in Ayurvedic medicine and Chinese medicine to improve digestion and clear out residue from the digestive tract.

- *Biotics Research HCL Plus®* is my favorite product, only available through health professionals. Because it contains two different acids, one to break the food down and the other to rehabilitate your stomach to make stomach acid.
- *Braggs Organic Apple Cider Vinegar®* is what I usually recommend because of the high quality and purity of the product. Generally one tablespoon at the beginning of a full sized meal is recommended.
- *Lemon-* just use the juice of a real lemon, there are lemon juices in bottles at the grocery store that contain chemicals and preservatives that are to be avoided. Use the same as you would vinegar or put onto bitter greens for an even better start to the meal.

Digestive Bitters are just like they sound, bitter! Don't expect them to taste good, but this is a necessary flavor to entertain. Remember you have four different taste buds to use. Bitters stimulate the secretion of stomach acid and stimulate bile flow out of the gallbladder thereby unburdening the liver. Your liver hangs onto medications, hormones, pesticides, cholesterol and more that it needs to release with the help of proper bile flow out of the gallbladder. Think of your gallbladder like a turkey baister, one good squeeze and it full, one good squeeze and its empty again. You want your gallbladder to empty, it's important. Here are a few of the brands of herbal bitters I recommend:

- *Gaia Herbs Sweetish Bitters®*
- *Eclectic Gentian Angelica Bitters®*
- *Flora Maria's Original Herbal Bitters®*
- *Angostura Bitters®-* these are basically 'bar bitters' used to make mixed drinks. Every restaurant with a bar has them, you can order a shot and drink no more than half the shot

glass to stimulate digestion. Especially important before a fatty meal.

Digestive Emulsifiers, such as Lecithin derived from soy, is a very useful and important supplement if the bile is too thick or sluggish. Your bile should contain emulsifiers, but if they don't get to mix with the food, then fats [a.k.a. cholesterol, hormones and vitamins] don't get managed properly. A simple lecithin capsule at the beginning of each meal can be very helpful.

- *NOW Brand Lecithin®* comes in granules, liquid and capsules. Any form will work, the capsules are just more convenient.

Digestive enzymes help to break food down if the stomach acid is weak or there are inadequate pancreatic enzymes. If the food does not break down properly, fermentation of the food in the digestive tract leads to formation of gas, alcohols and sugars that contribute to bloating, yeast/candida overgrowth, constipation or diarrhea, and inflammation of the tissue.

- *Metamorphosis Products Transformizyme™* is a broad spectrum digestive enzyme designed to break food down to very small particles so that food allergies and gluten doesn't get recognized by the immune system. For those of you who have Celiac, this doesn't mean you don't have to be gluten free, but the enzymes help in case there is gluten residue in your food.

Probiotics, also known as 'good bacteria,' are an important part of your immune system defense and without them you are more likely to become ill.[ii] Antibiotics destroy good bacteria in the gut and leave you vulnerable to other infections and yeast overgrowth. Yeast overgrowth contributes to carbohydrate cravings, weight gain, elevated blood sugar and liver congestion among other problems.

- *Metamorphosis Products ProBio Repair* ™ is an allergen-free, high potency probiotic useful for treatment after antibiotics, prolonged digestive problems or recovery from a severe illness.
- *Metamorphosis Products Pro Bio Maintain*™ is an allergen-free broad spectrum probiotic for everyday use that support natural amounts of good bacteria in the digestive tract.

6.   EAT ADEQUATE DIETARY FIBER

The digestive tract depends upon fiber to remain healthy. A mixture of soluble and insoluble fiber is necessary to achieve the normal shedding of old cells from the lining of the intestines, and the re-building of new cells. Insoluble fiber is rough and is meant to make the bowel movement move along and take away debris with it from the digestive tract. Soluble fiber is gooey and forms the proper size of a bowel movement while feeding the good bacteria along the way. The good bacteria secrete chemicals that renew cells in the intestinal lining and protect against inflammation.

To be specific, a normal bowel movement is approximately 6-8 inches long, about an inch in diameter, and medium to dark brown without mucous or blood. A normal bowel movement should be eliminated at least once and no more than three times a day. For those of you who don't look in the toilet, please start! This is an important way to know if your digestive health is on track.

With proper fiber in the digestive tract your body is able to make vitamin K, necessary for proper clotting and bone strength, and vitamin B12, only found in the animal kindgdom, in order to remain healthy. See Chapter 6: High Fiber Diet for all the details on how to achieve a healthy balance of fiber in your daily diet.

7. CONSULT WITH A HEALTH PRACTITIONER

If you are having any serious digestive issues, please seek evaluation from a health care professional. Most people avoid colon cancer screening out of fear of the preparation or wishful thinking it won't happen to them. Don't be one of those people- GET SCREENED!

Here are the symptoms to be most concerned about needing immediate attention and screening:

- Small, pencil like stools
- Bowel movements that are black or bloody not from iron, bismuth or iron rich foods
- Persistent abdominal gas, bloating or distention
- Abdominal pain, rectal pain, or pressure
- Inability to have a bowel movement daily
- Mucous or white film on bowel movements

Also seek the advice of your primary care physician to ensure you are screened properly for colon cancer risk:

- Colonoscopy beginning at the age of 50 unless family history indicates earlier screening
- Genetic testing if there is two or more colon cancers or melanoma in the family tree
- Examination immediately for any blood or change of bowel movements not related to dietary intake

DIGESTIVE HEALTH TESTING

Find a Naturopathic or Alternative doctor that conducts functional medicine testing to evaluate your digestive system. We use specialty laboratories to test for several digestive health markers:

- Levels of good bacteria, presence of unwanted bacteria, or yeast and fungal growth in excessive amounts
- Digestive secretion markers such as pH, pancreatic markers, bile markers
- Bowel wall health as indicated by the presence or absence of short chain fatty acids and inflammatory secretions
- Beta-glucuronidase is an enzyme that promotes the formation of cancer forming chemicals in the intestinal tract and has been linked with the formation of colon cancer and implicated as a risk factor for breast cancer. Elevated levels can be treated with the use of Calcium-d-glucarate supplementation, probiotics, high fiber diet, proper digestive pH, and vitamin C to lower the risk of cancer formation. Testing is available through Genova laboratories.

WHAT TO DO: Have a screening colonoscopy by the age of 50. Begin a digestive enzyme at the beginning of each meal and a probiotic at bedtime. Obtain a medical evaluation for any digestive problems that persist or require the use of over-the-counter medication on a regular basis.

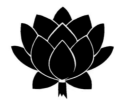

Chapter 2:
Optimizing Food Quality

Now that you have strong digestion, it is important to select the highest quality foods available. I want you to become a food snob and demand the best! First, you have to learn the good and the bad of what is available at the grocer. There is a lot of misleading news about organic foods in particular, so I will very simply inform you. I am asking you to learn the facts for yourself and use common sense to decide what you will purchase or eat from here forward.

The U.S.D.A. labels organic products with their seal of approval (see below). If a food says "organic" but does not have this seal of approval, then it is likely from another country that does not carry these standards and cannot be trusted as a truly organic food.

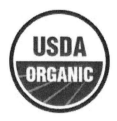

ORGANIC FOODS

When you buy organic, you are not only making a choice about the food you are eating, you are making a choice about which industry to support and how you want the environment to be treated in the process.

What goes into a food being labeled organic?[iii]

- The land for the animals or plants has to be toxin-free
- The feed for the animals has to be toxin-free
- The water for the animals or plants has to be toxin-free
- The living conditions for animals has to be health promoting
- The growing conditions for plants has to be disease resistant and the soil nutrient-rich
- No harmful drugs or pesticides can be used in the growing process, which also protects our drinking water supply
- Farmers must keep detailed records, have their farms inspected, and have written Organic Plans detailing their farming management practices in order to be certified as an organic farm.

Some small farms use organic practices but do not get certified because the fees are exorbitant for level of profits. In contrast, non-organic farming practices use methods that are more concerned with volume and production rather than our health or the environment and are the main contributors to polluted water ways and nutrient-stripped land masses.

When it comes to commercial animal food production, the most revealing information on the meat industry is found at www.peta.org. Many animals are not raised in a healthy manner and are slaughtered in filthy and inhumane conditions. Contaminants in the meat include hormones, bovine-growth hormone, and pesticides from non-organic feeding practices, antibiotics from infections that fester from poor living conditions, adrenaline and stress hormone from the stressful living and slaughtering conditions, chemicals used to treat the tainted meat before it is sold, and possibly the feces of the animal that has contaminated the meat. These drugs and chemicals are harmful to the human body and do not show up on the label when you buy your meat, but you get them when you buy commercial meat.

When it comes to the environment, commercial animal farming is a large consumer of fossil fuels, introduces chemicals and drugs into local water supplies, creates excessive methane gases and manure disposal issues, contributes to the worldwide problem of antibiotic resistant bacteria, consumes excessive amounts of water compared to produce production, and undermines or drives out smaller farmers with better farming practices.[iv]

Non-organic produce crops absorb one-third to one-half of the chemical fertilizers applied, less than 1% of the pesticides reach the pests they are intended for, and all of these chemicals pollute the surrounding waterways. Pests have developed resistance to these chemicals and pesticides and their use has been linked with honey-bee population death.[v] Pesticides have also been associated with cancer development, reproductive problems, and behavioral abnormalities.

So, do you really want to keep buying non-organic foods? How about planting a garden in your backyard or on your patio this year? Why not plant a kitchen herb garden to use year round? These measures can only help you so far, and then you have to decide what to buy at the grocery store. You can become a member of a natural food buyers' co-op, or crop share with local farmers, or use the space at community gardens. Find out what is available in your local community so you can plan ahead for the next year on how to improve the quality of your food supply.

FOOD LABELING, INGREDIENTS & PACKAGING

After selecting your organic meat, dairy and produce, then you have to decide what else to consider purchasing. If you are going to use processed or packaged foods, then you need to learn how to read the ingredient list, decipher the label claims and know how food is packaged in order to avoid an onslaught of toxins in your body from the food you eat.

All
Natural

Natural- There is no formal regulation of "natural" labeling on food products and the definition is whatever the word itself implies. Our expectation is that the food was grown naturally without pesticides and that there are no 'bad' things added. This is not necessarily true since the word "natural" is completely unregulated. According to the Food Marketing Institute, the label of "natural" is applied to foods that are minimally processed and free of synthetic preservatives; artificial sweeteners, colors, flavors, and other artificial additives; growth hormones; antibiotics; hydrogenated oils; stabilizers; and emulsifiers. The FDA, however, only restricts the use of the term on products that contain added color, synthetic substances and flavors. The rest is up for manufacturers to admit to using or not.

WHAT TO DO ABOUT BUYING "NATURAL"? Read the ingredient list for additives, preservatives or chemicals and as long as you recognize the ingredients as real and not artificial, then consider it for purchase.

Wild Caught vs. Farm Raised fish- Data on salmon, specifically, indicates that farm raised clearly is not the same quality as fish caught from the wild. Farm raised fish presents environmental issues and may have parasites, inadequate omega 3 oils, a higher concentration of inflammatory producing oils, and a higher pesticide, toxin and heavy metal content.[vi]

WHAT TO DO ABOUT FISH?- Make sure it is wild caught or responsibly farm raised, know the country of origin, do not get pre-seasoned packaged fish varieties, and check these websites for additional information:

http://www.wholefoodsmarket.com/products/aquaculture.php

www.seafoodsafe.com

www.safeharborfoods.com

 www.aquaculturecertification.org

Country of Origin- Not all countries have the same growing standards making your food source an important food fact to know about. Sometimes imported foods may say "organic," but they are not unless they are certified organic by the USDA. Single sourced food items, such as meat, dairy and produce need to be labeled with country of origin. Food items with multiple ingredients do not have to list the country of origin, and then you don't know what they did to the food.

In 2007, the Associated Press put out an article on the safety and quality of imported foods. Their findings discovered infrequent food inspections, tainted food, poisons, and revealed that food safety experts have admitted that the US cannot ensure the imported food supply is safe. [vii] You have to ask yourself "What is in my food that I don't know about?" I'm sure that you and I don't really want to know, but it does force you to think about where you food is coming from.

The UPC code is where the final product is being sold from and that is where the bar code originates so it is a very difficult task to know the origin of your food! There is conflicting information about how to read a bar code to determine country of origin and the following information is likely the UPC code prefixes for certain countries:[viii]

00 ~ 13 USA & CANADA
30 ~ 37 FRANCE
40 ~ 44 GERMANY
49 ~ JAPAN
50 ~ UK
57 ~ Denmark

64 ~ Finland
76 ~ Switzerland and Lienchtenstein
471~ Taiwan
628 ~ Saudi-Arabien
629 ~ United Arab Emirates

690-695-China
740 ~ 745 – Central America

All 480 Codes are Made in the Philippines.

Additives, Preservatives, & Excitotoxins- There are many food chemicals allowed into the food supply that are considered safe, but there is growing controversy in the food industry as to whether or not that is really the case. Just ask Dr. Russell Blaylock, author of *Excitotoxins: The Taste that Kills*, who can attest to the dangerous ramifications of food manufacturing chemicals entering the human body. [ix] Dr. Feingold, founder of The Feingold Diet, also dedicated his professional life to helping children with behavior and developmental problems to become well again by removing harmful food chemicals from the diet.[x]

I have had many patients over the years that improved with removal of food additives alone. One case that stands out in my mind was a woman who presented with progressive weakness, was walking with a cane, was out of work on disability, and had a negative work-up for Multiple Sclerosis and Lyme disease. When questioned about any diet product use, she admitted to using artificial sweeteners in her food plus a liter of diet soda a day! Within three weeks of stopping these artificial sweeteners, she was walking without a cane and more oriented than she was at the first visit. Case after case of neurological and behavioral problems, including migraines and ADHD, improve after stopping artificial food additives.

Here are some of the most problematic food additives:

- *Monsodium glutamate (MSG)*- an amino acid flavor enhancer, contributes to migraines, is a known contributor to neurological problems, can cause severe allergic reactions, seizures, heart rhythm disturbances, and is believed to contribute to obesity, metabolic syndrome and diabetes.[xi] As it stands right now, there are no regulations requiring the listing of MSG as an ingredient in a product so you are literally taking your chances when you are eating any processed food unless the manufacturer goes to the point of saying MSG is not in the product.

- *Potassium bromate*- an oxidizer used in commercial flours, is known to interfere with proper thyroid function due to inhibition of iodine, and is a carcinogen in animal studies, mainly associated with renal cell carcinoma. According to the Center for Science in the Public Interest, even though a cancer risk was identified in 1991, the FDA only urged bakers to stop using it rather than banning its use altogether.[xii] Potassium bromate is in nearly every baked good that you buy at the grocery store.

- *Disodium EDTA*- EDTA is commonly used in food and beverages as a preservative and stabilizer and protects food products from discoloration and oxidation. EDTA reacts with Vitamin C (ascorbic acid) and sodium benzoate in sodas and bubbly drinks, forming benzene, a known carcinogen.[xiii]

- *BHA & BHT [Butylated Hydroxyanisole and Butylated Hydroxytoluene]*- they are questionably carcinogenic (cause cancer) and can affect behavior and the nervous system according to Dr. Feingold's work. [xiv]

- *All synthetic food colorings/dyes*- animal research has shown it may be linked with causing cancer, yellow dyes in particular are a known trigger for asthma attacks, and all food dyes are considered excitotoxins that over-stimulate the nervous system.[xv]
- *Sodium benzoate*- I already noted that sodium benzoate and vitamin C form benzene that is a known cause of cancer. In addition, Dr. Piper from Sheffield University reported in 1999 that sodium benzoate interferes with mitochondrial DNA, the place in your body that makes energy for your muscles to move.[xvi] Basically this ingredient makes you want to sit on your behind and not go exercise, a huge contributor to obesity among other things like fibromyalgia and chronic fatigue! Sodium benzoate is a preservative in all soft drinks and some junk foods and candies.
- *Sodium nitrite/nitrate*- when you eat these chemicals, nitrosamines form in the stomach and can contribute to the development of cancer, specifically stomach cancer and brain tumors. Even if you choose nitrite & nitrate free deli products, they contain celery juice in place of chemicals, but the same harmful chemical is formed by the interaction of the nitrites in celery and the bacteria of the meat, so you are not really any better off. Cured meats are just going to be a problem not matter how you slice it [pun intended!].
- *Sulfites*- this is a big topic that I am going to distill down [again, pun intended!], that includes wine, beer, vinegars, dried fruits, preserved foods and frozen dinners as likely sources of sulfites. If you have a sulphur drug allergy or asthma, you are not likely to not tolerate sulfites and can develop a rash, congestion, or wheezing. For all the rest of us, we may tolerate them but to varying degrees. Sulfites are

measured in part per million, not labled as such, and are only noted on some food products as "Contains Sulfites."

- ***Trans-fats*** - primarily found in the form of hydrogenated vegetable oil contributing to heart disease and abnormal blood lipid levels. See Chapter 8: Omega-3 Balanced Diet
- ***Artificial Sweeteners*** - See Chapter 5: Low Glycemic Diet

"Use By" or "Sell By" Dates-There is not a universally accepted expiration date labeling system for the US food supply except for infant formula and some baby foods. If a date is present, then obey the date on the package for freshness.

Food Packaging Toxin Exposure- In 1995 the United States banned the use of lead solder in cans. But lead solder can still be found in cans made in other countries. These cans usually have wide seams, and the silver-gray solder along the seams contains lead which over time gets into the food. Cans containing lead may be brought to the United States and sold. Once the can is open, the lead leaches faster, especially with acidic foods.[xvii]   Lead is a known toxin to the nervous system and main contributor to abnormal cognitive development in children.

Bisphenol A (BPA) is the main component of epoxy resin food container liners that prevents the food from reacting with the metal. BPA is believed to be a hormone disruptor and is ubiquitous in our food supply of all packaged foods. The most concerning exposure is for babies during pregnancy that can change how the estrogen receptors function for the rest of their lives.[xviii]

Since the first announcement of BPA-related health problems in 2008, major food suppliers have been attempting to convert their food packaging to become BPA-free. According to a recent article in the Washington Post, providing BPA-free food with new packaging materials may be more challenging than first thought.[xix]

What the Bleep $#@! Can I Eat?

The article reports that Eden Foods, an organic food manufacturer that switched to BPA-free food packaging, had traces of BPA in their beans according to an independent testing agency. They also mention the same scenario with Vital Choice Tuna. Sprout Organic Baby Food also provides food I BPA-free packaging, but it is likely they face the same challenges along with all the other companies trying to succeed in this arena.

FOOD STORAGE AND PREVENTING SPOILAGE

Now that you have purchased the best meat, dairy and produce that you can find, you want to store them in a manner to prevent spoilage. Modern refrigeration is an ally for optimal food storage with buttons for each bin temperature. Even with that, I find that buying produce more than three days in advance is usually a disappointing scenario. Food has already traveled in trucks across the country many days after being picked and packaged and has sat in grocer's refrigerators spoiling. The best approach is to shop twice weekly for perishable food items and select the best looking ones available at the store.

Begin with buying only a few delicate produce items and plan to eat them within the first two to three day s after purchase. The hardier produce, like the broccoli family, will last much longer. Asparagus, celery, and scallions can all be stored vertically in a glass with water in the bottom. The same technique can be used with herbs, just snip off the bottom of the stems and place in a water glass.

Ethylene gas is emitted from ripening fruits and vegetables, the more gas released, the faster the ripening of the produce. There is a gadget called the "E.G.G., Ethylene Gas Guardian," that absorbs ethylene gas in your produce bin and prevents premature ripening of fruits and vegetables. The E.G.G. is available at most health food stores or online.

The rest of your storage depends upon using your refrigerator the way it was designed. Read your manual to see where it is best to store meat, dairy, and produce to maximize the shelf life of your perishable foods. Also learn how to use any levers for the bins to set the humidity or temperature correct to prevent spoilage.

Natural bread poses its own challenges because there are no preservatives. Bread will keep on the counter for a day or two, then into the fridge for a day or two and then you will have to freeze the rest. The shelf-life of bread will depend upon which brand and the climate of your kitchen, but most importantly, the lack of artificial preservatives that prevent mold growth.

Nuts and seeds should be treated like perishable food items because of the delicate oils they contain. Once a nut is outside of its shell it is vulnerable to rancidity. Nuts and seeds should be stored in airtight containers, in a cool cabinet, or preferably in the refrigerator. Use them within three months and discard the entire batch if there is any visible mold growth or tainted odor coming from them.

Dry goods and grains can potentially introduce pantry moths into your kitchen. Preventing an infestation is easier than eradicating the flying critters. Vacuum out your kitchen cabinets, wash them down with a vinegar-water solution, and store whole grain products in sealed containers [especially from bulk bins at the health food store!]. Whole grains and flours can be stored in the freezer overnight prior to putting them into the pantry as a measure to kill any larvae they may contain. Long term storage of grains and flours is not recommended without proper nitrogen packing equipment to ensure freshness and prevent meal moths.

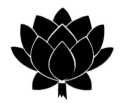

Chapter 3:
Allergen-Free Diet

You may already know you are allergic to certain foods from having been tested or suspect that you are based on symptoms that you are having. I will give you an idea of how to proceed based on the type of allergen or sensitivity you are having and you can learn how to avoid the most typical allergens in your daily diet.

There are common allergenic foods that are fondly referred to as the 'sinister seven' which include dairy, wheat, corn, citrus, soy, peanut, and egg. In part, these foods have become popular allergens because they have been over-consumed and our immune systems are basically saying "No More!" Since these foods are the ones people often eat, they are the same ones that are sorely missed when removed from the diet. First, learn whether or not you can temporarily remove the food or whether you should avoid it all together by getting tested.

IgE allergies tend to be stubborn and the reaction more intense, sometimes even dangerous. Immediate histamine allergies (IgE type) can produces hives, swollen lymph nodes or mucous membrane swelling in the sinuses, throat, airway, stomach or intestines. In the worst case, anaphylaxis can develop which affects the breathing from swelling in the airway leading to loss of consciousness. IgE allergies are either realized by the patient having a reaction or detected by routine blood allergy panel testing. Food avoidance, antihistamines, and possibly the need to carry an Epi-pen are typically how these are treated. Sometimes even a minor exposure to the food can cause serious reaction, therefore, consult with your health care practitioner to determine how strict your avoidance efforts need to be.

Delayed food reactions (IgG), referred to as "sensitivities", can cause a problem within minutes of eating or up to three days after. Symptoms may include migraines, stomach ache, rashes, eczema, bed wetting, seizures, digestive problems, or itchy skin. Sensitivities are difficult to detect by food journaling because the time span for reactions is so broad. I recommend specialty laboratory testing to detect these food reactions. Reactive foods are then eliminated from the diet for a period of a few months. Additional testing is done approximately two to three months later to determine that the digestive tract is healed. If healing is complete, the foods are reintroduced one at a time to see if they can be tolerated without a reaction. Many times patients don't even realize how badly they felt until foods were eliminated and reintroduced. If the food is well tolerated, a rotation diet is adopted where the food item is limited to every 3-4 days.

In addition to immune reactions, wheat and dairy contribute to mucous formation which is problematic for asthmatics or anyone with sinus congestion problems. Whether you are allergic to them or not, whenever you are congested, it is best to avoid wheat and dairy until the illness has passed.

DAIRY AVOIDANCE

Dairy avoidance obviously includes milk, yogurt, cheese, butter, cream and ice cream. The more challenging avoidance is to foods that are prepared with dairy as an ingredient. Hidden dairy ingredients may be listed as casein, lactose, lactalbumin, whey, recaldent (in chewing gum & dental products), Ammonium caseinate, Calcium caseinate, Casein hydrolysate, Iron caseinate, Magnesium caseinate, Paracasein, Potassium caseinate, Rennet casein, Sodium caseinate, and Zinc caseinate.

Dairy milk, both cow and goat, contains more calories, protein and fat than any of the vegetarian milk substitutes. Goat milk products may be the best substitute for cow milk products because of its nutrient content and possibly lower risk of allergy. According to one source, "Goat milk contains only trace amounts of an allergenic casein protein, alpha-S1, found in cow milk. Goat milk casein is more similar to human milk, yet cow milk and goat milk contain similar levels of the other allergenic protein, beta lactoglobulin. Scientific studies have not found a decreased incidence of allergy with goat milk, but here is another situation where mothers' observations and scientific studies are at odds with one another." [xx]

It is especially important to consider calories, fat and protein intake for children with food allergies for proper growth and development. The taste of goat products, however, may take some getting used to, and they may not necessarily be any less allergic.

Many look to soy as their first option as a dairy substitute. One of the problems is that soy is also one of the 'sinister seven' foods to be avoided, unless you have been tested and know it is not an allergen. Most allergy panels include soy, so check your results. Also, not all soy is necessarily beneficial.

Milk & Substitutes 1 cup	Calories	Protein	Fat	Carbohydrates	Additives
Cow Milk	146	8	8	13	Vit A, D3
Goat Milk	168	9	10	11	---
Soy Milk	130	8	3.5	18	---
Rice Milk	120	1	2.5	23	Vit A, D2, B12
Almond Milk	40	1	3	2	Vit A, D2, E
Hemp Milk	60	1	6	1	Vit A, D2, B12 Riboflavin

Fermented forms of soy such as tofu, tempeh, miso and natto have the least amount of phytic acid that interferes with mineral digestion, most importantly zinc, iron and calcium necessary for proper growth and development. Eden Foods has an entire article on their website dedicated to how their food production technique lowers the phytic acid content of their products, specifically their soymilk, making it a healthy part of the diet as compared to other commercial brands.[xxi]

There are also concerns with unfermented soy because of the hormone disrupting isoflavone diadzein. Genestein, the preferred isoflavone more prevalent in fermented soy products, has protective benefits on reproductive tissue and bone health.

Other dairy substitutes are often high in carbohydrates, lack beneficial fats, and do not provide an acceptable amount of protein, calories or nutrients to be considered a true 'substitute' for milk. You may also find dairy ingredients listed in these products such as casein or whey. Your best reassurance is when the product is labeled "vegan" it will not contain any animal sourced ingredients.

While dairy does have lactose sugar, it has protein and fat to offset the ill effects of sugar to some extent. Many people are lactose intolerant and find they have to use lactose-free options. Lactose intolerance can be tested for and often eliminated as a problem when we work on optimizing disgestive health (see Chapter 2: Optimizing Digestion). Yogurt contains very little if any lactose and can be used plain to avoid any simple carbohydrates from dairy all together. Choose unsweetened varieties of dairy substitutes and be very selective about which sweeteners you will use in your diet. This will be covered in greater detail in Chapter 5: Low Glycemic Diet.

Another problem with dairy substitutes is that they often contain polyunsaturated fats that contribute to omega fat imbalances in the body. Polyunsaturated fats are believed to contribute to development of cancers and cardiovascular disease because of their ability to promote inflammation and are best to be avoided. Read your labels for safflower, corn, sunflower, cottonseed, and soybean oil as ones to avoid as much as possible. See Omega-3 Balanced chapter for more details.

WHEAT AVOIDANCE

Wheat, like dairy, can be found in many prepared food products. Wheat is in baked goods, cookies, crackers, breads, pastas and used as binders or thickeners in processed food. You have to expand your thinking to recognize everything that is made from wheat. White bread is really wheat, kamut and spelt are wheat, semolina flour in pasta is wheat, cous cous is pasta (wheat) cut into little pieces, and tabouli is made with bulgur wheat.

Wheat avoidance is definitely challenging! Hidden wheat ingredients may be found listed as bran, wheat germ, farina, gluten, graham flour, gluten flour, protein flour, vital gluten, gluten, malt, wheat starch, modified food starch, hydrolyzed vegetable protein, natural flavoring, soy sauce/tamari, vegetable starch or vegetable gum. Also refer to the extensive list of gluten ingredients in the next chapter, but by no means do you have to convert to a gluten-free diet based on this allergen alone.

Wheat alternatives include all grains and starches that are not derived from wheat. Rye and barley products contain gluten, so if you are Celiac, then these have to be avoided as well. Corn is considered a grain, but is one of the 'sinister seven' allergies and is best to be avoided if you haven't been allergy tested. Otherwise, the best wheat alternatives are quinoa, oats, amaranth, buckwheat (which is not wheat at all), rice, potatoes, and arrowroot. There are many wheat-free food products available as well, however, they may contain gluten or corn so read your labels carefully!

CORN AVOIDANCE

Eliminating corn from your diet is usually prompted by allergy testing. Most patients who have tested positive for corn allergies were unaware of this as the culprit for their symptoms. Corn avoidance can be equally as challenging as wheat and dairy because the food industry uses corn derived ingredients in so many food products.

Corn oil, corn syrup solids, modified food starch, corn starch, baking powder (contains starch), possibly caramel, confectionary sugar (contains cornstarch), dextrin, maltodextrin, dextrose, fructose, glucona delta lactone (in cured meats), invert sugar/syrup, malt, mono/di-glycerides, sorbitol, and anything made with corn are to be avoided. Breaded foods often contain cornmeal in the mix and pizza can have cornmeal on the bottom of the crust. Sometimes you have to call the food manufacturer to see if their ingredients are derived from corn or not, such as corn maltodextrin.

Corn avoidance is difficult because it is often the replacement ingredient in wheat-free or gluten-free processed foods. Avoiding corn is best achieved by cooking from scratch by simply avoiding the corn products. Arrowroot is the replacement for cornstarch and works just great in recipes. Baking powder contains cornstarch and can be made from scratch using ½ teaspoon cream of tartar + ¼ teaspoon baking soda. Corn syrup can be replaced with equal amount of maple syrup or honey in recipes. You can even make your own confectionary sugar, since it usually contains cornstarch, by adding 1 ½ Tablespoons of tapioca or potato starch to 1 cup granulated sugar and process in a high speed blender for 45-60 seconds until powdered.

CITRUS AVOIDANCE

Many times patients have already figured out they don't tolerate citrus because of prickling in the mouth, a rash around the lips, canker sores in the mouth, upset stomach and sometimes cystic acne. Citrus allergy can be detected by conventional and specialty lab testing as well.

Citrus avoidance includes oranges, lemons, limes, grapefruit, clementines, tangerines, kumquat, and mandarin oranges. Citric acid is added as a preservative to many processed and packaged foods including juices and fruit products, vitamins, medicines and candy products.

If you prepare foods from scratch then avoiding citrus should not be difficult. Otherwise, you need to read ingredient lists carefully for foods containing citrus juice or citric acid preservatives.

SOY AVOIDANCE

The good news is that soy nearly matches dairy for calories, protein and fat which makes is a good dairy substitute, as long as you're not allergic to it. The bad news is that a lot of patients really are allergic to soy and don't realize it. Testing is a good idea in this case, especially if you are vegetarian and this is your main protein source.

Soy foods include soymilk, soy yogurt, soy kefir, soy cheese, soy ice cream, soy cream cheese, tofu, tempeh, miso, soy sauce/tamari, and meat substitutes made with soy protein. Soy is often used in processed vegetarian foods and everything from soup to frozen meals and burgers. Soy is also in most of your popular protein bars as the main source of protein.

Soy can be hidden in food and listed as soy protein, soybean oil, soy sauce, soy curd, soy flour, soy grits, soy nuts, soy milk, soy sprouts, isolated soy protein, soy protein concentrate, hydrolyzed soy protein, textured soy protein, soy meal, soy isolate, soy isoflavones. Soy oil and lecithin are less problematic because there is essentially no protein to react to making them neutral to keep in the diet.

Because soy is a member of the legume family, those with food intolerance, allergy or sensitivity to soy should watch carefully for reaction to other legumes such as peanuts, chickpeas, lentils, black beans, and other kinds of beans. If there is a true allergy to soy, then the legume family may also have to be avoided. Again, this is problematic if you desire to be vegetarian so testing is your best guide on which foods to avoid.

PEANUT AVOIDANCE

This is usually the food allergen that gets all the attention because of how severe the reaction can be. Peanut IgE allergy requires you to carry an Epi-pen and stay in the "peanut-free zone" as is dedicated in many cafeterias. IgG peanut allergy or sensitivity is a delayed reaction that is less severe and does not require such alarm. Peanut sensitivity may cause symptoms in the digestive tract, sinuses, or skin as well.

Attention Pregnant Women:

Avoid all peanut products in an effort to reduce or eliminate the risk of severe peanut and other food allergies in the baby!—Dr. A

Peanuts will always be listed as on label as peanuts, peanut oil, or "made in a facility that processes peanuts". Grocery shopping for peanut-free is relatively easy if you just read the labels. Restaurant dining, however, poses greater challenges since peanut oil is used in many kitchens because it is inexpensive, can tolerate high heat, and is desirable in many ethnic dishes due to its distinct flavor.

Substitutes for peanuts are easy to find because of the variety of nut products on the market. Nut butters and nut oils of every variety are readily available. These products, however, are not always produced in a peanut-free facility which is a concern for those with severe IgE allergies to peanuts.

EGG AVOIDANCE

Many patients have already figured out they are allergic to egg by virtue of the reactions they get after eating egg. Typically gas, bloating, stomach pain, and skin rashes can be attributed to egg allergy or sensitivity. Testing can be very helpful in determining whether to keep egg in your diet or eliminate it completely.

What the Bleep $#@! Can I Eat?

Globulin, albumin, apovitellenin, livetin, ovalbumin, ovomucin, ovomucoid, ovovitellin, phosvitin, are food ingredients derived from egg. Whole eggs, egg whites, egg yolks, dried eggs or egg powder, and egg solids are all obvious ingredients to avoid as well.

Keep in mind the foods that are made with egg. For example, most everything battered has egg, Ceasar dressing and creamy dressings have egg, Chinese mu shu and mai fun are cooked with scrambled egg, many noodles and pastas contain egg, many ice creams have egg, and even Snickers bars have egg! Egg wash may also be used on pretzels. Read your labels!

For baking, there are powdered 'egg substitutes' available at the health food store. They are a bit difficult to use at times and work best if you mix it swiftly and add it in at the last minute before putting your batter in the pans. Instead, you can try substituting any of these options for the equivalent of one egg:

½ tsp. baking powder + 2 tablespoons water

1 T. ground flax seeds + 3 T. water + 1 T. oil + 1 tsp. baking powder + 1 tsp. arrowroot

¼ tsp. agar agar + ¼ c. water + 1 tsp. baking powder

¼ c. banana or other fruit puree (doesn't always work, experiment!)

Tofu is a good substitute for egg as a scramble, in potato salad, in quiche, cream pies, in meatloaf or meatballs, and many other dishes as long as you are not allergic to soy. Manufacturer recipes or vegetarian cookbooks may be your best resource on which type of tofu best suits your recipe.

What the Bleep $#@! Can I Eat?

ALLERGY-FREE FOOD BRANDS

There are certain companies that cater to having allergen-free foods available. You still have to read labels and see the ingredients to suit your specific needs, but it does narrow down the search! My best advice to you is begin shopping at the health food store, then look for those brands at your grocery store or buyers warehouse. Once you know what is available, it makes your life a little easier! Keep in mind that prepared and canned foods often have too much sodium added so choose the low salt or no salt options whenever possible. I have starred (*) my favorite choices for quality, nutrition, versatility and/or likability:

- Schar*- bread products, pizza crust [has corn & soy]
- Sunshine Burgers*- they have a good amount of protein without the use of soy or egg
- Amy's Organic*- chili, soups, meals [some have soy]
- Bob's Red Mill*- bread mix, soup mix, hot cereal mix
- Mary's Gone Crackers*- whole grain crackers and cookies
- Suzie's*- rice thins
- Vance's Dari-Free- milk and cream alternatives
- Rice Dream- milk, ice cream
- Mimic Cream- instant coffee creamer
- Purely Decadent- coconut based milk, ice cream
- Food for Life- bread products, read labels
- Diamond Nut Thins- crackers
- Orgran products- read ingredients
- Enjoy Life- bars, granola, cereals
- Ener-G- egg replacer
- Ancient Harvest*- quinoa products, some contain corn
- Tinkyada*- pasta products
- Hodgeson Mill*- rice pastas

- Roads End- gravy mixes, mac & 'cheese'
- Erewhon- cereal products
- Miss Robins- baked goods and mixes, read ingredients
- Hol-Grain- Tempura mix and Breading mixes
- Glutino- snack foods, bread products
- Breads from Anna- yeast free, allergen-free mixes
- Eden Organics*- beans, milk substitutes, read ingredients
- Imagine Soups*- read ingredients for different flavors
- Lundberg*- read ingredients
- Coconut Secret Non-Soy Sauce
- Vegennaise- egg-free mayonnaise
- Galaxy Foods- vegan dairy alternatives
- Living Harvest*- hemp milk
- Applegate Farms*- meat and deli products (sparingly)
- Natural Sea- canned tuna without vegetable broth (sparingly)

ALLERGEN-FREE MEALS

One thing is for sure, being picky is not a good character trait if you have to adopt an allergen-free diet! You have to bring your sense of adventure and trust me when I say it gets easier with time. One consideration is that allergies in general rob you of zinc, and zinc is responsible for the taste buds liking lots of flavors and colors in the food. Sometimes we have to supplement with zinc just to get the taste buds to cooperate for introducing new foods!

The other aspect to adopting an allergen-free diet is that you need to keep this simple enough to manage, but have meals taste good enough that you will be happy eating. In the beginning, you are better off cooking very plain, simple meals until you stock-up your kitchen and find some items that you like. For some of you these changes are temporary for three or more months, for others this may be a lifelong change you need to make.

Keep notes, save package wrappers, and shop at different stores until you find what you need. Lastly, don't kid yourself into thinking you can avoid your allergen just some of the time and cheat the rest of the time. You really have to eliminate the allergen completely to begin the healing process which takes months, and get tested or advised by your doctor when you can reintroduce that particular food item again.

Allergy-Free Breakfast Options

#1: Chicken sausage, sautéed vegetables, potato hash (recipe to follow)

#2: Oatmeal with rice protein added, almonds (or suitable nut/seed), berries, raw local honey, and cinnamon

#3: Bob's Red Mill Rice Hot Cereal with rice protein added, walnuts, blueberries, maple syrup and cinnamon.

#4: Black beans, salsa and guacamole on a rice tortilla wrap

#5: Sunshine Burger Breakfast Pattie, Schar multigrain toast, strawberries

#6: Applegate Farm Turkey bacon, sliced tomatoes, red onions and Food for Life English Muffin (gluten-free, egg-free, corn-free, dairy-free)

#7: Minute steaks with onions and mushrooms, over baby spinach and Schar multigrain toast, berries on the side

Allergy-Free Lunch Options

#1: Chicken or turkey over a salad, Bragg's Vinaigrette dressing, and hummus on Suzie's rice thins (remember that deli meat requires reading all the ingredients, best to grill/bake it yourself).

#2: Salmon or white fish made into a cold salad with Vegennaise, served on Schar bread with leaf lettuce, sliced onions, sliced tomato and raw vegetable sticks, and a cup of bean soup (Amy's Organic-read ingredients especially for corn)

#3: Eden Beans & Quinoa (can), green salad, guacamole on Suzie's rice thins

#4: London broil slices, spinach strawberriy salad with Bragg's Vinaigrette, and rice crackers.

#5: Amy's Vegetarian Chili, baked potato, and salad

#6: Personal pizza with Schar crust, Muir Glen Pizza sauce, toppings of choice, Vegan Rice Mozzerella and a salad

#7: Sunshine Burger, Schar Bun, sliced tomato, onion, and leaf lettuce. Serve with sweet potato fries.

Allergy-Free Dinner Options

Dinner is easier because you are home and can prepare the meal from scratch. You may even need to keep some frozen dinners with the ingredients you need for when you are in a hurry or need to eat outside of the home when visiting others. Just be aware of sodium content in these packaged food items.

First, pick your protein and decide how you want to cook it. Second, select a hypoallergenic grain such as rice, quinoa or pasta. Lastly, add vegetables either steamed or raw to go with it.

What the Bleep $#@! Can I Eat?

#1: Chicken- stir-fried, baked, or grilled with wild rice or Lundberg Risotto, and steamed vegetables

#2: Turkey- ground turkey as tacos or burgers, or roasted turkey breast, quinoa, and steamed vegetables

#3: Fish- baked, with basmati rice and steamed vegetables

#4: Steak- London broil, organic or natural, baked potato, green beans

#5: Beans- Vegetarian chili (Amy's Organic, Eden bean mixes), whole grain such as quinoa/brown rice and steamed veggies

#6: Tinkyada Spaghetti & Turkey Meatballs made with gluten-free breadcrumbs (no egg or cheese in the balls)

#7: Pizza as above for lunch with sautéed greens

French Toast

Milk or milk substitute in a shallow dish/bowl, add vanilla bean or extract, and cinnamon. Dip one piece at a time of bread before placing in skillet with melted coconut oil. Lightly brown on each side, serve with maple syrup, breakfast turkey pattie, and fresh berries. You can make batches of French Toast and freeze it for future use.

Hotel Salmon Breakfast -My favorite!

This is a great substitute for those of you who like to get cream cheese on a bagel and call it a breakfast. Only now you will get protein, omega-3's, antioxidants, and whole grain fiber without any allergens. Hooray!!!

Nitrite-free Smoked Salmon on Food for Life Whole Grain Gluten-free English muffin with country Dijon mustard, sliced red tomato, sliced red onion, a sprinkle of dill and optional capers. Serve with fresh blackberries and a small amount of vegetable juice. All that color and flavor is wonderful!

Cold Fish Salad Sandwich

Canned tuna, salmon, or crabmeat [read can for "broth" which contains MSG and/or wheat] drained and flaked into bowl, add minced onion, celery, parsley, Celtic Sea Salt and ground black pepper. Add Vegennaise to bring the mix together. Serve on a gluten-free English muffin or bread. Optional to melt cheese on top and serve as a traditional tuna melt. Serve with wedges of tomato or cup of tomato soup [Imagine brand] and a pickle [Cascadian Farm].

Chicken Fajita Wrap

In a skillet, lightly sauté slice onions and peppers, add raw or previously cooked chicken, add Frontier Organics Taco Seasoning, a squeeze of lime juice, and wedges of tomato. Place into brown rice or corn tortilla with guacamole. Serve with black beans and rice.

Make Your Own . . .

For nights when you have no energy or time, or when you have to appeal to lots of different people's taste preferences or allergies, have a "Make Your Own" night. Great for birthday parties or when the kids have friends over.

- Burritos with Spanish Rice and steamed vegetables
- Tacos with Beans & Rice and salad
- Open Faced Sandwiches with Soup and Cooked Greens
- Personal Pizzas with Broccoli Raab/Salad/Green Beans

Fillings can be Amy's Beans, or Turkey Meat with Frontier Organics Taco Seasoning, or Shredded Chicken with Taco Seasoning and diced tomatoes. Topping for sandwiches can be pastrami, corned beef, turkey, chicken, turkey bacon, sauerkraut, vegan cheese, and soup from Imagine. Pizza topping can be gluten-free BBQ sauce with chicken; Mediterranean veggies such as calamata, roasted peppers, artichokes, olive oil and garlic; or just Muir Glen Pizza sauce with whatever vegetables you like.

Allergen-Free Snack & Dessert Options

Here is where all the trouble begins because I know this is probably the first place people go to find their relief from all the stress of eating allergy-free. The problem is going to be finding foods that are not highly refined with a lot of sugars added. It is very difficult to find whole grain, wheat-free options. These are some choices that are available. **Please know that eating fresh fruit, vegetables, nuts and seeds are actually the better choices for snack foods compared to some of these options:**

- So Delicious Coconut Ice Cream
- Barbaras Wheat-free Fig Bars
- Mary's Gone Crackers- crackers and cookies
- Enjoy Life Bars
- Suzie's Rice thins with hummus, nut butter, or guacamole
- Nut-Thins with hummus
- Mochi puff pastry filled with bean spread, nut butters or guacamole- they are divine and very filling!

What the Bleep $#@! Can I Eat?

ALLERGY-FREE RESTAURANT DINING TIPS

Wait staff are trained better than ever to help you experience allergy-free dining. If you have multiple allergies, it is best to write them down on an index card and keep it in your wallet for use when ordering. An allergy-free website will create your communication card called "Allergy Buddy Card." Enter your request to "supermarket guru" at: http://archive.supermarketguru.com/page.cfm/7512 to get your card and get started. Another site called "allergy free passports" has books to help you travel and eat out, apps for electronic handheld equipment, and even translation cards in other languages for foreign travel. Go to www.allergyfreepassport.com for apps.

Some restaurants are becoming known for their ability to accommodate those with food allergies and have been noted by national news articles for their efforts. Ask for an allergy-free menu when being seated, many of your major chain restaurants now have these available. Here are a few restaurants with allergy-free menus available that I am aware of:

- Boston, *Blue Ginger*
- Chicago, *Bistro 110*
- New York, *Babycakes Bakery*- this one you have to check out!
- Ruby Tuesday's
- Olive Garden
- Outback Steakhouse
- T.G.I.F.
- Macaroni Grill

So all it takes is some testing, some reading and some special shopping to get you on the road to good health. Eventually you may be able to add back in the allergenic foods, but follow the advice of your health care practitioner based on your test results and symptoms you are trying to avoid. An unapproved or premature binge or splurge could land you in the hospital with a bowel obstruction among other problems. That's exactly what happened to one of my patients when he decided it was time to have some pizza on a Friday night. Two pieces of pizza and 24 hours later, he was regretting that decision!

PARENTS OF CHILDREN WITH FOOD ALLERGIES

As a parent, you will likely be able to spot a food infraction in your child when their eyes look glassy, lips appear red, or they are congested, itchy or running to the bathroom more often. All allergies need to be clearly reported to school nurses, teachers, day care providers, grandparents and babysitters. Most people do not understand how vigilant they need to be at reading labels and sometimes think that a little cheating won't hurt.

One suggestion I give to parents of children with food allergies is to develop a food package notebook where you place the actual packaging of allowed purchased foods inside of plastic page protectors. You can also create a master grocery list of brands and specific foods that caregivers can keep on hand if they will be giving your child meals or snacks. This is especially important for grandparents who seek the rewards of love and affection from your child by giving out treats. Provide caregivers with healthy snacks so they can have options that don't harm the child's health.

Lastly, be aware of the volume of food the child is eating and whether or not they are growing and developing properly. You need to make every effort to provide adequate nutrients and calories while avoiding the allergenic foods. Height & weight should be monitored no less than every three months to make sure the child is receiving enough nutrients. Consult with your child's health care provider to monitor.

FOOD ALLERGY RESOURCES

Living Without magazine and website provides multitudes of recipes for commonly sought out foods that people miss when they avoid allergenic food. This is an invaluable resource for beginners.

NavanFoods website- allergen-free shopping at its best! This website has most everything you need to find to get started. Use this site to at least make your initial grocery list- narrow your choices by searching by your dietary restrictions, then scroll down and see what your options are. It's terrific!

U.S. Biotek Food Allergy Testing- is an affordable fingerstick test that evaluates IgG sensitivities of foods and optionally spices & herbs. Results come with a booklet to guide you with allergen avoidance. Test needs to be ordered by a health care professional.

Genova Laboratories Intestinal Permeability Testing- is a urine test to determine if the gut is allowing food particles to leak across the membrane or if malabsorption of nutrients is occurring, both are often linked with food allergens.

Allergy Free Passport.com to get apps for your phone or portable device to assist you in finding allergy-free dining establishments.

Food Allergy and Anaphylaxis Network- www.foodallergy.org. This is a great website for specific categories of allergens including fish, shellfish, tree nuts, and peanuts.

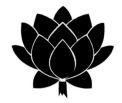

Chapter 4:
Gluten-Free Diet

Many patients ask if they would benefit from a gluten-free diet. My advice to them is that if they have symptoms that can be related to gluten, first get tested before going gluten-free. Adopting a gluten-free diet when medically indicated is not usually a temporary measure. At some point you are going to second guess being gluten-free and testing is the determining factor which should be done while you are still eating gluten.

Symptoms may include abdominal pain, diarrhea, constipation, eczema, cough, headache, joint pain, rashes, weight problems, hyperactivity, and more. The cliché symptom of Celiac disease is diarrhea, but my patients have shown me a multitude of symptoms and nutrient deficiencies that lead to investigating for Celiac. In my opinion, this is currently one of the most overlooked diseases in pediatric medicine [vitamin D deficiency is the other].

Celiac Disease, A.K.A. Celiac Sprue, is a genetically inherited autoimmune reaction against gluten that damages the small intestine and prevents nutrients from being absorbed. The diagnosis of celiac requires the complete and long-term removal of gluten from the diet. When celiac goes untreated it leads to malnutrition, osteoporosis, skin disorders and a greater risk of developing lymphoma in some individuals.

Why is it so important to know if gluten is a problem even if it's not Celiac? You want your immune system and body organs well functioning. The small intestine can become inflamed and dysfunctional leading to key nutrient deficiencies such as fat soluble vitamins (A, D, E, K), B vitamins, Iron and amino acids. These are all necessary for proper growth and development of children and for the prevention of many major diseases that our society suffers from today.

The most reliable testing is done by blood testing for IgE allergy, IgG sensitivity and celiac screening. In my opinion, relying on muscle testing (kinesiology) or electronic testing to adopt a gluten-free diet is just not definitive enough. At some point you're going to second guess the diagnosis and not know what the real problem was. I also take into account the patient's nationality, family history and the symptoms of the patient to help them decide whether or not to have a patient become gluten-free.

IgE testing can be done for wheat, rye, barley and gluten to determine if gluten grains cause a histamine allergic reaction. Symptoms tend to be more immediate and dramatic. This is typically managed by food avoidance, homeopathic desensitization, and possible reintroduction if the food is tolerated without symptoms or an increased serum IgE level.

IgG sensitivity testing is typically done through a specialty lab and detects a different part of the immune system that becomes active against wheat, barley, rye, gluten or gliadin. Symptoms can occur within hours or up to three days later making them difficult to identify with simple food journaling. These results lead to an allergy elimination diet and possible eventual inclusion of the food on a limited basis as part of a rotation diet.

Celiac laboratory screening looks for anti-gliadin antibody, anti-endomesial antibodies and tissue transglutaminase. In my opinion, if any of these are positive, then it's time to go gluten-free and document what symptoms resolve as a result of the diet change. All too often patients have already been screened by a physician prior to my evaluation and have been told they were "negative" for Celiac. When I obtain copies of labwork and find any elevated readings, the outcome is ALWAYS a positive one for the patient when they remove gluten from their diet.

On occasion, the testing proves negative but the patient is convinced that they react to gluten grains or the family history is so positive that it warrants testing for the Celiac gene. HLA typing for Celiac is conducted, and in my opinion if it is positive, then the person should consider themselves affected by Celiac. When my patients in this category become gluten-free, they ALWAYS report positive outcomes!

Unfortunately, the gastroenterology community is focused on scoping and biopsying to make a confirmative diagnosis. Even those with a negative biopsy have benefited from becoming gluten-free in my practice. This is a complicated and multi-factorial problem. Our genes have been bombarded by gluten over the generations and our bodies are saying, "Enough!"

Additional testing may be necessary once a gluten problem has been identified. Blood counts, chemistry panels, and vitamin testing should be done as a baseline to determine what nutrients must be supplemented while healing takes place. It can take months and up to a year to recover proper function of the small intestine once becoming gluten-free.

What the Bleep $#@! Can I Eat?

I do not prescribe a gluten-free diet lightly! Both my children and I are gluten-free and it is one of the hardest things we have had to do as a family. But when I think back to all the colic, green diarrhea, yellow frothy bowel movements, variable appetite, rashes, red bumps, and mood changes, going gluten-free is worth it!

Once you are told to become gluten-free, you should go 'cold turkey' off gluten. There is no wiggle room to keep a little in the diet. First you need to learn what gluten ingredients look like. The following list shows the many ways gluten can be hidden or included in food products.

GLUTEN INGREDIENTS TO AVOID OR INVESTIGATE

Abyssinian Hard (Wheat triticum durum)
Amp-Isostearoyl Hydrolyzed Wheat Protein
Atta Flour
Barley Malt
Beer (contain barley or wheat)
Bleached Flour
Bran
Bread Flour
Brown Flour
Bulgur
Cereal Binding
Chilton
Club Wheat (Triticum aestivum subspecies compactum)
Common Wheat (Triticum aestivum)
Cookie Crumbs, Dough
Couscous
Crisped Rice
Durum wheat (Triticum durum)
Edible Coatings, Films, Starch

Einkorn (Triticum monococcum, dicoccon)

Farina, Farina Graham

Farro

Filler

Fu (dried wheat gluten)

Germ

Graham Flour

Granary Flour

Groats (barley, wheat)

Hard Wheat

Heeng

Hing

Hordeum Vulgare Extract

Hydrolyzed Wheat Gluten, Protein, Wheat Starch

Kamut (Pasta wheat)

Kecap Manis (Soy Sauce)

Kluski Pasta

Maida (Indian wheat flour)

Malt, Malted Barley Flour, Milk, Extract, Syrup, Flavoring, Vinegar

Macha Wheat (Triticum aestivum)

Matzah

Oriental Wheat (Triticum turanicum)

Orzo Pasta

Pasta

Pearl Barley

Persian Wheat (Triticum carthlicum)

Perungayam

Poulard Wheat (Triticum turgidum)

Polish Wheat (Triticum polonicum)

Rice Malt (if barley or Koji are used)

Roux

Rusk

What the Bleep $#@! Can I Eat?

Rye
Seitan
Semolina, Semolina Triticum
Shot Wheat (Triticum aestivum)
Spirits (some)
Spelt (Triticum spelta)
Stearyldimoniumhydroxypropyl Hydrolyzed Wheat Protein
Tabbouleh/Tabouli
Teriyaki Sauce
Timopheevi Wheat (Triticum timopheevii)
Triticale X triticosecale
Triticum Vulgare (Wheat) Flour Lipids, Germ Extract, Germ Oil
Udon (wheat noodles)
Unbleached Flour
Vavilovi Wheat (Triticum aestivum)
Vital Wheat Gluten
Wheat, Abyssinian Hard triticum durum
Wheat amino acids
Wheat Bran Extract
Wheat, Bulgur
Wheat Durum Triticum
Wheat Germamidopropyldimonium Hydroxypropyl Hydrolyzed
Wheat Protein
Wheat Nuts
Wheat Protein
Wheat Triticum aestivum
Wheat Triticum Monococcum
Wheat (Triticum Vulgare) Bran Extract
Whole-Meal Flour
Wild Einkorn (Triticum boeotictim)
Wild Emmer (Triticum dicoccoides)

GLUTEN-FREE PACKAGED FOODS

Food products are considered "gluten-free" if they contain less than 20 parts per million (ppm) of gluten accordancing to current Codex limits for naturally gluten-free food. Codex is a joint effort between the Food and Agriculture Organization of the United Nations and the World Health Organization and sets the standard of gluten content allowed in a food product labeled to be gluten-free. The trap is to buy "gluten-free" foods, but they are not necessarily the healthiest foods and tend to be VERY expensive! In the end, let simplicity win out and prepare foods simply from scratch for the most enjoyable, healthy, and economical outcome!

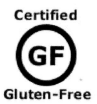

Thankfully there are many gluten-free foods on the market. Gluten-Free food labeling can now be certified through The Gluten Free Certification Organization (www.gfco.org). This group inspects products for gluten content and is the only company offering this certification to food companies as an opportunity to better market their products. Keep in mind, the process is voluntary and business driven, so the food company is motivated to have the label and the certifier is motivated to sell the label. All the other foods on the market labeled "Gluten-Free" is without any verification by any organization. However, there are standards in the field as to how the kitchen or facility needs to maintain the environment to prevent contamination.

GLUTEN-FREE KITCHEN

So, how do you manage a gluten-free household? Does everyone have to become gluten-free? The answer is a little complicated. First, consider what foods and equipment are being used in the kitchen. If you are using a lot of flour products in the kitchen that result in flour dust covering surfaces, then converting to a gluten-free kitchen is desirable to avoid cross-contamination. You may need to get rid of some kitchen equipment, for example we used to make homemade pasta, but we had to get rid of our pasta maker, drying racks, and pizza stone since they cannot be completely cleaned of gluten flour residue. However, getting rid of the toaster oven may be going overboard for most cases. In some respects, having a gluten-free kitchen is like having a kosher kitchen, the gluten items need to be kept separate.

If the rest of the household has been tested and can have gluten, then it is a practical reality that they will have gluten grains in some capacity. Making the adjustments to include a gluten-free family member just takes a little adjustment. For example, the gluten-free pasta is drained in the colander before using it to drain the gluten pasta. Gluten-free toast is toasted prior to gluten toast and then the racks are cleaned before the next use. Gluten-free food items can be expensive and best used on the person who needs them the most. You also have to reserve a place on the grill just for the gluten-free items for marinades, etc. to not be contaminated.

GLUTEN-FREE PANTRY

One of the challenges with gluten-free prepared food is the lack of nutrients such as B vitamins and fiber. Patients with Celiac are usually already B vitamin deficient, so this is undesirable from a nutrition standpoint. Many of the choices are white and starchy and are not well suited to those with hypoglycemia, diabetes, obesity or high cholesterol. There are some products that deliver a better quality product because they use the whole grain, but they are few and far between. I have tried what I believe to be nearly every popular GF item at typical health food stores, and there is a short list of what is most desirable.

These are a few of my favorite things to keep in the pantry and freezer (if you can imagine me singing this to you like in the sound of music! ☺):   [GF=GLUTEN FREE]

Tinkyada- GF Organic Brown Rice Pastas

Hodgeson Mill- GF Brown Rice Pastas, Pancake Mix

Lundberg- GF Brown Rice Couscous, Risotto mixes

Food Merchants- GF Quinoa Polenta

Orgran- GF Falaffel Mix

Mary's Gone Crackers- GF Original Flavor Crackers

Suzie's- GF Brown Rice Thins

Schar- Multigrain Bread

Food for Life- GF Multiseed English Muffins

French Meadow Bakery- GF Flour Tortillas

Mission- GF Corn Tortillas

Bearitos- taco shells and seasoning

Bob's Red Mill- GF All Purpose Baking Flour

What the Bleep $#@! Can I Eat?

Bob's Red Mill- GF Biscuit and Baking Mix

Arrowhead Mills- Blue Cornmeal

Orgran- GF Buckwheat Pancake Mix

Lifestream- GF Buckwheat Waffles

Natures Path- GF Mesa Sunrise Cereal

Enjoy Life- Perkeys Crunchy Rice or Flax Cereal

Enjoy Life- Cinnamon Crunch Granola

Udi's GF Granola

GF Rolled or Steel cut Oats

Ancient Harvest- GF Quinoa Flakes

Bob's Red Mill- GF Mighty Tasty Hot Cereal

Stop trying to cook with gluten-free mixes, and start thinking how to cook from scratch. Virtually every meal made from scratch does not need to be complicated if you use some of the gluten-free staples above with it. Once you get into buying all the different starches and flours, things get pretty messy and less healthy! The feedback I get from patients is that they are tired of baking and making gluten-free foods and that buying commercial products is expensive. But when asked if they have plain grains they cook from scratch, the answer is usually "No." Stock up on the basic staples and you will do just fine.

GLUTEN-FREE MEALS

Gluten-free Meal Construction:

- Choose a protein first- chicken, turkey, fish , beans, tofu, egg
- Choose a fruit or vegetables suitable for the meal
- Select a food starch such as potatoes or rice, or use one of the gluten free food products on my favorites list
- Use olive oil, apple cider vinegar, lemon juice, real herbs, organic spices or sea salt for seasoning

Breakfast Options

#1: Eggs, GF toast/English muffin, berries

#2: Yogurt, GF granola, berries

#3: Salmon, GF toast/English muffin, tomato & onion, berries

#4: Turkey pattie, potatoes, green apple slices

#5: Almonds, GF oats, blueberries

#6: Peanut butter, GF waffle, strawberries

#7: Chicken sausage, Buckwheat pancakes, mixed berries

Lunch Options:
#1: Hardboiled eggs on a salad with Mary's gone crackers or egg salad w/vegennaise on Schar multigrain bread and veggie sticks

#2: Black beans, spinach, red pepper, corn and salsa on a salad or in tacos, or on top of polenta

#3: Grilled chicken on a salad with quinoa tabouleh on the side

#4: Turkey burger, potato salad w/vegennaise, vinegar green beans

#5: Cold Fish Salad either on top of a salad or in a rice flour wrap with lettuce, with carrot sticks and cucumber spears

#6: Cold macaroni salad: make a little extra macaroni at dinner the night before, add a protein (chicken, fish, tofu, beans), add 1 cup frozen mixed vegetables (thawed in colander) and toss in vinaigrette dressing. Serve the next day for lunch with tomato soup and rice crackers.

#7: GF Falaffel, hummus, carrot sticks, and cucumbers with yogurt and dill on top

Dinner Options:

#1: Baked fish, brown basmati rice, mixed vegetables all sprinkled with toasted black seasame seeds and a drizzle of gluten-free sesame teriyaki from Organicville.

#2: Grilled chicken, Lundburg Parmesan Rissotto, Broccoli raab in olive oil and garlic

#3: Baked turkey tenderloin, gravy (Roads End), organic cranberry sauce, pumpkin, and green beans w/almond, olive oil and lemon juice

#4: Grilled London Broil (organic, natural), A-1 Steak sauce, steamed red potatoes with olive oil and crushed garlic, broccoli and salad

#5: GF Amy's Chili over baked potatoes served with cooked greens, olive oil and garlic

#6: Crustless pizza (see recipe below) or a gluten-free pizza, escarole with olive oil, garlic and white beans

#7: Scallops pan seared in olive oil, with artichoke hearts, sundried tomatoes and calamata olives over gluten-free pasta served with lightly steamed asparagus in olive oil and lemon juice

GLUTEN-FREE ITALIAN DINNER FEAST

- GF Breadsticks (Schar, Glutino) served standing up in a glass
- GF Antipasto- greens, Applegate farm salami and provolone, Mediterranean organics roaster peppers and artichoke hearts
- Olive dish- Mediterranean organics variety olives
- White Bean and Escarole soup using GF Imagine Chicken broth as the base
- Stuffed shells using ricotta, pure pecorino romano, and parsley as the filling, Tinkyada shells, organic pasta sauce, and organic shredded mozzarella for the top
- Dessert Assortment: Mariposa biscotti, organic gelato, fresh berries, nuts in the shell and organic coffee

GLUTEN-FREE INDIAN DINNER FEAST

- GF Poppodums (Tiger Tiger)
- Chicken Masala (breasts or thighs, Ethnic Gourmet Calcutta Masala sauce and simmer)
- Mixed Vegetable Korma (1 bags of Cascadian Farm California Blend frozen vegetables, 2 medium potatoes cubed, 1 can garbanzo beans, drained, Ethnic Gourmet Dehli Korma sauce and simmer)
- Jyoti lentil dahl
- Jyoti Peas & Paneer Cheese

- Basmati Rice
- I like to serve a mint sauce or cucumbers with yogurt and mint as a side dish as well.
- Dessert possibilities: Gluten-Free Rasgulla based on a sweet fluffy milk base (recipe available on website www.bookofyum.com), Gluten-Free Modaks are rice and coconut steamed dessert dumpling (recipe available on website www.thecolorsofindiancooking.com), or just chew on a few fennel seeds to sweeten your breath.

GLUTEN-FREE THAI DINNER FEAST

- Rice Paper Spring Rolls (see recipe below) with Thai Peanut Satay (A Taste of Thai)
- Amy's Coconut Thai soup
- Pad Thai (chicken, shrimp or tofu)- follow package instructions for rice noodle preparation, stir-fry the protein with onions, red peppers, baby corn, green onions, add the noodles, and pad thai sauce (A Taste of Thai, Tasty Bite)
- Curried vegetables (1 frozen bag of Cascadian Farm California Mixed Vegetables, 4 Potatoes, 1 can Thai coconut milk, Frontier Organic Curry Powder, Celtic sea salt to taste)
- Dessert Option: Toasted Coconut Fortune Cookies (A Taste of Thai)

GLUTEN-FREE MEXICAN DINNER FEAST

- Organic tortilla chips and organic salsa and Wholly guacamole
- Bearitos Taco shells, taco seasoning with turkey, buffalo or tofu

- Taco toppings of lettuce, tomato, black olives, and organic
- Near East Spanish Rice
- Amy's Organic Refried Beans

GLUTEN-FREE DESSERT OPTIONS

This can be a little tricky. The first priority is making sure the mixes or ingredients are gluten-free. Many people don't know they have to read the ingredient list for specific chemical names of ingredients such as maltodextrins, gums, and natural flavorings. Always ask to see the list of ingredients when eating something that has been pre-made by someone else. Also, consider what the kitchen environment is where the baked goodies were made. Your gluten-free goodie could be contaminated with gluten flour! Bummer, I know!

If you are looking for goodies for the kids, and sometimes for the grown-ups, then there are many options. On the one hand, there are more choices available than ever, on the other hand, they remain an expensive indulgence. You are always better off with fruit, nuts, seeds and the like, but I thought you would want to know about the other fun foods. I have purposefully included choices that also do not have harmful food chemicals, additives, and aim to have healthy ingredients. If you search the internet for gluten-free food lists, you will find a list of commercial products, but that doesn't mean they are healthy or even should be included in your choices.

Here are some ideas on treats that are gluten-free:

- Gluten-free ice cream on a gluten-free cone with gluten-free sprinkles
- Luigi's frozen lemon ice- a good one to keep in mind when the ice cream truck rolls through the neighborhood.
- Minute Maid frozen fruit pops, no artificial dyes

- Breyer's All Natural Ice Cream (lactose-free vanilla available) with fresh fruit
- Ben & Jerry's has a list gluten-free of their gluten-free ice creams (not all of them have the best ingredients)
- Andean Dream Gluten-Free (allergen-free, vegan) cookies-great ingredients!
- Cherrybrook Farms Mixes for gluten-free chocolate chip cookies, brownies, and cakes (not only gluten-free but egg & dairy-free as well)
- Schar- has a variety of cookies, virtually the Pepperidge Farm of gluten-free goodies! They even make gluten-free Ladyfingers to make Tiramasu! [I am going to work on a recipe for a gluten-free, egg-free, dairy-free Tiramasu and will post it on my website when I have perfected it!]
- Enjoy Life- cookies, bars, snacks
- Kinnickinick- variety of cookies, does contain egg.
- Mariposa Biscotti- these are definitely worth a try with some tea or coffee!
- Nana's cookies- can be egg free, dairy free as well.
- Orgran- variety of fun shaped cookies, great for toddlers and younger kids.
- Grainless Baker- they actually have gluten-free graham crackers (also Kinnickinick), an essential ingredient for S'mores when kids go to camp. Send along with gluten-free marshmallows (Campfire brand) and an organic chocolate bar.

EATING GLUTEN-FREE WITH FRIENDS & FAMILY

You can be included in gatherings by keeping food prep simple. Just inform your host that you can't have any seasonings or sauces, to cook things from scratch, and pick from the categories below:

- Eggs, Tofu, Chicken, Fish, Egg or Beans for protein
- Rice, corn, potatoes, or GF oats for starch
- Vegetables and fruits, raw or lightly steamed, without marinades or sauces

Keep things simple! Families that try to use gluten-free mixes, etc. usually get themselves into trouble in the kitchen! Explain that you don't need baked goodies and special breads unless they are truly up for the challenge. Most of the bread mixes are white, starchy, and lack adequate vitamins or fiber. Also, in most cases the bread machine needs to be dedicated to just gluten-free mixes.

DR. A'S FAVORITE LITTLE GLUTEN-FREE DISHES

Crustless Personal Pizza

1 boneless chicken breast per person, hammered thin, misted with olive oil, baked on cookie sheet at 425° for 20 minutes until mostly cooked. Spread Muir Glen pizza sauce, add whatever toppings you like, top off with shredded mozzarella cheese, put it back into the over for another 10 minutes to cook the toppings and you've got pizza! What's nice about this recipe is that you can order your meal this way at restaurants and not miss out on dining out for Italian with friends and family.

Rice Paper Spring Rolls

Oriental rice spring rolls, as many as you want, soak in warm water before stuffing to make them pliable. Stuff by placing a pile across the center using thin pieces of food such as beef, chicken, tofu, scallions, peppers, zucchini, yellow squash, bean sprouts, shredded carrot, and bok choy or lettuce. Fold over the edge perpendicular to your pile, then fold over each side piece. Dip into oriental sauce such as Organicville sesame teriyaki or Annie Chung sauces (check labels).

Muffin Cup Crustless Quiches

Using coconut oil, grease the cups of a muffin tray. Using a glass pitcher, whisk together one egg per muffin cup plus a splash of cold water until frothy. Place the following items into each empty muffin cup: torn baby spinach, chopped onion, pepper/tomato, and shredded cheese (optional). Pour the egg over the ingredients in each cup. Bake at 350° until the eggs puff up and you get a clean toothpick from the center, approx. 20 minutes. Take out of the oven, let cool so that tops flatten, then remove from muffin tray. Serve for breakfast or with a nice salad for lunch. These will keep well in refrigerator for at least two days and heat up well without being rubbery, so don't be afraid to make a big batch!

Parchment Pouch Meals

One of my favorite ways to cook is with the use of parchment paper pouches. They retain all the nutrients of the food, but also keep foods from touching each other. Each pouch contains just what the person wants and there are no problems with cross contamination. Basically, you wet the parchment paper with water, place food items in the center, fold and tuck in ends, coat with oil, and place on the grill. The pouches steam and cook within 20 minutes for most meals. This keeps food allergens from touching one another and there are no pans to clean up in the kitchen!

Peaches and Cream Dessert

Fresh peaches, halved and pitted, and lightly grilled on either side or lightly steamed. Mix fresh vanilla bean with ricotta cheese.

Arranged grilled peach halves on plate, fill with a scoop of Ricotta, drizzle with raw local honey, and sprinkle with grated dark chocolate or crushed coffee bean and a sprinkle of organic cinnamon.

Fresh Berry Pie with Nut Crust

Using a food processor, grind 1 ½ cups of nuts (walnuts & pecans), then add 4-6 pitted dates, 2 pitted prunes, a sprinkle of cinnamon and 1-3 tablespoons of water or any juice to create a dough. Press into a glass pie dish. You can either fill it as is or bake it at a low temperature for 20 minutes to firm up. Fill with fresh berries, yogurt, ice cream and berries, pudding and berries, or basically whatever you want and refrigerate or freeze it until serving. My husband is the pie maker in the house, and the pumpkin pie is to salivate over! Consider whipped coconut milk using arrowroot as a thickener.

TIPS ON CONVERTING A RECIPE

- Baking- use Bob's Red Mill All Purpose Flour in place of the flour requirement
- Asian cooking- use wheat-free tamari and arrowroot instead of soy sauce or other thickeners
- Italian cooking- replace pasta with gluten-free pasta, bread mixes from Bob's Red Mill, Namaste, Gluten-free Baker

DETECTING GLUTEN IN FOOD

Trying new products or eating out can be challenging and worrisome. Elisa-Tek is a testing company that sells gluten testing strips to determine if any gluten is in the food you are about to eat. The test will detect as little as 10 ppm and has proved its worth in detecting gluten in foods that are labeled "Gluten Free" that actually weren't. The disadvantages to using these test strips is that each test costs about $25 and it takes 10 minutes to process making it impractical for daily use. Test strips are available at www.EZGluten.com.

GLUTEN-FREE DINING

The good news is that restaurants are catching on to meet the needs of the ever-growing gluten-free community. Outback Steakhouse, Ruby Tuesdays, Olive Garden, and many pizza restaurants are now providing gluten free pizza and pastas. For gluten-free restaurant participation, you can check the website of The Gluten Free Restaurant Awareness Program at www.glutenfreerestuarants.com and look up one in your area. If you want to travel, there are gluten-free vacations as well. Check out www.celiactravel.com or www.glutenfreetravelsite.com. There are many different gluten-free websites and resources so you won't feel alone on this food adventure!

Gluten-free eating can be challenging and complicated, so the best thing to do is to KEEP IT SIMPLE. Just eat 'real' food whenever possible, as opposed to processed and packaged food, that way you don't have to worry about what is in your food and your grocery bill won't be outrageous. You will find that friends and family want to come to your aid, just be discerning about what they have to offer you. Keep in mind that "gluten-free' is not completely regulated and that ultimately you have to read the list of ingredients. Be well and enjoy!

GLUTEN-FREE RESOURCES

www.celiac.org Celiac Disease Foundation

www.celiac.com Informational website

www.glutenfreeliving.com Gluten-free Living Magazine

www.glutenfree.com Online shopping for gluten free foods

www.glutenfreetravelsite.com For gluten free vacations

Also keep in mind that almost all of the gluten-free food manufacturers have recipes and helpful information directly on their websites. There are also local Celiac support groups for closer, ongoing support with your path to health.

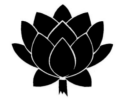

Chapter 5:
Low Glycemic Diet

Everyone can benefit from a low glycemic diet. Consider this as
your first defense against three of the most common causes of death
and disability in adults- cancer, diabetes and heart disease! Blood
sugar levels over 120 begin to affect the immune system in a
negative way. Under normal circumstances, white blood cells need
vitamin C to phagocytize (eat up) viruses, bacteria and cancer
cells.[xxii] Sugar looks similar to vitamin C and enters the cell instead
rendering the white blood cell useless until it can receive the vitamin
C.[xxiii] Maintaining blood sugar levels normal (under 99) allows your
white blood cells to survey for infections and cancer properly.[xxiv]
Lastly, there is even growing evidence that vitamin C-sugar
competition is a contributor to cardiovascular disease, commonly
found in diabetics.

If you have diabetes in your family history or if you are overweight,
fatigued, over-stressed or sedentary, then you need to have your
blood sugar markers evaluated. Ask your doctor for a fasting blood
sugar, insulin, IGF-1, hemoglobin A1C, lipid panel and AM cortisol.
If you also suffer from symptoms of hypoglycemia such as weakness
or shakiness if you miss a meal, then you should also receive a three
hour glucose tolerance test with insulin at every draw. In my

practice I have patients aim to keep their fasting blood sugar less than 90, insulin below 10, IGF-1 in normal range, HA1C below 5.7, triglycerides <130 and AM cortisol between 15-20. The glucose insulin tolerance test will illustrate if there is reactive hyper or hypoglycemia and insulin resistance. Anyone who has abnormal results is prescribed a low glycemic diet.

Metabolic Syndrome is the diagnosis given to people with abdominal obesity, hypertension, insulin resistance, and glucose intolerance. There is a growing population with this syndrome attributed to a lifestyle full of stress, inactivity and poor dietary habits. In my practice, the biggest excuses for not eating well are "not enough time," "too tired, " "too lazy," and "overeat when upset or stressed." The low glycemic diet must be considered like a dose of medicine for those with Metabolic Syndrome because their lifestyle is working against them and inevitably leads to diabetes, heart disease and possibly cancer.

A low glycemic diet corrects hypoglycemia, insulin resistance, pre-diabetes, diabetes, high triglycerides, high cholesterol, obesity and adrenocortical stress by stabilizing insulin levels and blood sugar. There are two methods to evaluating foods the hurt or help blood sugar, Glycemic Index (GI)and Glycemic Load (GL), to guide you on which foods to include in your low glycemic diet.

The Glycemic Index (GI) is a numerical Index that ranks carbohydrates based on their rate of glycemic response (i.e. their conversion to glucose within the human body). GI uses a scale of 0 to 100, with the higher value given to foods that cause the most rapid rise in blood sugar. Pure glucose serves as a reference point with a Glycemic Index of 100. The lower the GI, the better your control of blood sugar and insulin levels.

Low GI: 55 or less

Medium GI: 56-69

High GI: 70+

Glycemic Load (GL) was first popularized in 1997 by Dr. Walter Willett and associates at the Harvard School of Public Health. Basically, foods that contain high dietary fiber have a low GL because fiber slows down the glucose from entering the bloodstream. Glycemic Load is calculated as follows:

GL= GI/100 x Net Carbs

Net Carbs: Total carbs minus dietary fiber

Low GL: <10

Medium GL: 11-19

High GL: 20+

Examples of Low Glycemic Foods

	GI	GL
Blackberries	32	4
Blueberries	40	6
Raspberries	32	3
Strawberries	32	3
Grapefruit	25	5
Cherries (tart)	22	7
Walnuts	18	0
Coconut, raw	10	1
Pine nuts	10	0
Artichoke	20	3
Asparagus	15	2
Broccoli	15	2

Brussel sprouts	15	3
Cabbage	15	2
Cucumber	15	1
Lettuce, romaine	10	0
Red Pepper	15	3
Zucchini	10	2
Turnips	30	2
Green beans	30	4
Fish (most)	0	0
Egg	0	0

Instead of referring to charts or calculating food formulas, it's more important to understand the nature of food that makes it low glycemic. 'Simple carbohydrates,' namely sugar, white flour and pasta, are highly glycemic because the sugar can easily reach the bloodstream. Whole food carbohydrates such as brown rice, sprouted bread, steel cut oats that are lower glycemic than their refined counterparts because they contain valuable fiber.

Refined foods tend to be low in fiber as compared to whole foods which retain all their natural goodness including fiber and oils. The closer your food is to its original source, the more nutritious and the lower glycemic that food becomes. In the end, it's not just about blood sugar, it's about your overall health and wellness. Not only do you need to control the type of carbohydrates you eat, but also the volume and frequency of how you eat them.

One particular dietary caution, low-fat food items are often loaded with added sugars and salts. Conversely, low-carb foods often have harmful soy protein and loads of saturated fats. These notions are marketing tactics for selling you processed food shortcuts.

Glycemic Values of Refined compared to Whole Foods

	GI	GL
White Rice	64	33
Brown Rice	55	23
Popcorn	72	7
Corn, whole	54	9
Carrots, cooked	92	4
Carrots, raw	47	2
Quick Oats	94	17
Steel Cut Oats	42	17

Meals are best constructed by focusing on a lean protein, a small amount of plant fat, a fruit or vegetable, and small amount of grain every three hours. **Choose <u>one of each line item</u> to create a balanced meal:**

Breakfast:
- 3 egg whites/½ cup Greek yogurt/3 oz. fish or turkey meat
- ½ cup berries with ground flax seeds/ drizzle of coconut milk
- 1 slice sprouted grain toast- Ezekiel, Alvarado Street

Lunch:
- 3 oz. chicken/turkey/fish
- 2 cups leafy greens/cooking greens
- ½ cup beans/3/4 cup bean soup
- 1 whole grain WASA bread/Ryvita cracker/Ezekiel wrap or pocket
- 1-3 teaspoons olive oil/hummus/guacamole

Dinner:
- 3 oz. chicken/turkey/fish
- 1 ½ cup steamed non-starchy vegetables

- ½ sweet potato with a peel or brown basmati rice
- 1-3 teaspoons of olive oil/ nut oil

Snack Options for mid-morning or mid-afternoon:
- 1 T. nut butter on Suzie's brown rice thin/grannysmith apple
- 1 T. guacamole and fresh vegetable sticks
- 2 T. hummus and fresh vegetable sticks

I can hear you asking, "But what about dessert, popcorn, applesauce, etc…" I can tell you that there isn't a patient of mine who became well again eating these foods on a regular basis.—Dr. A

Even though ice cream is considered low glycemic (because of the fat content), it isn't a food I'm going to recommend because it doesn't contribute to health in any fashion, it is an inflammatory trigger causing pain, it raises cholesterol, contains harmful refined sugar, and directly causes obesity which is epidemic in our society! Stop looking for these types of sweets!

Here are some healthy dessert ideas to try:
- Steamed apple/pear topped with Bob's Red Mill muesli, serve with greek yogurt and a sprinkle of ground flax seeds and cinnamon
- Lightly grilled peach halves, fat free ricotta, a drizzle of honey, a sprinkle of cinnamon and a little shaved dark chocolate or crushed coffee bean sprinkled on top
- Mango pureed with lime juice layered with nuts, a sprinkle of ground flax seeds and a drizzle of honey [optional] in parfait cups
- Berries, drizzled with Thai coconut milk, a sprinkle of fresh

vanilla bean, grated fresh lemon zest, garnished with lemon balm or mint

One Note for Diabetics: Diabetics adopting a low glycemic diet should follow their blood sugars carefully and only reduce medication dosages under the supervision of their prescribing doctor.

SWEETENERS: FRIEND OR FOE?

In general, if you keep sending sweet signals to your tongue you continue to signal the part of the brain that craves the sugar. People crave sugar for a variety of reasons including emotions, fatigue, irregular eating patterns, and family history of alcoholism. The most important thing is to recognize your pattern and plan for success. Once you stop eating sugary foods, you may experience a sense of withdrawal and emotional upset. This is perfectly normal so just drink water, keep active and don't sit around the kitchen. The craving will pass after about three days.

Don't keep candy, soda, ice cream, cookies or foods like this in your house. Don't fool yourself into thinking you need to serve sweet desserts to company, they don't need it either! Stop kidding yourself by having a diet soda with a cheeseburger and fries as if you're helping yourself. Refined sugars and artificial sweeteners are addicting to the taste buds and the nervous system. Natural sweeteners from plants are not as addicting but must be used sparingly to keep the flavors in balance. It's time to change how you view food and retrain your body to not want added sweets.

NATURAL SWEETENERS

Natural, organic foods in their original state always have something beneficial to offer the body whether it is a vitamin, mineral or organic complex that improves some aspect of health. Even though these natural sweets may be beneficial, they must be used in small occasional amounts and should not be relied upon as a constant source of taste bud entertainment!

Raw Local Honey- A good batch of honey is like a fine vintage of wine! Those busy bees do a great job of making natural medicine that helps prevent seasonal allergies and boost the immune system! Once this golden nectar is heated, some of the benefit is destroyed, so just a fresh drizzle on top of what you are eating for the best use. Our honeybee population is suffering right now and we need to be mindful and grateful for the wonderful gift of honey!

Active Manuka Honey- Manuka is honey on steroids! This super power honey is getting all the attention for treating Helicobacter pylori stomach infections, Methycillin Resistant Staph (MRSA), Strep infections and more. There are even bandages now made with this honey!

Keep in mind, Active Manuka is in limited supply and should only be used like a prescription. I shudder at the thought of this honey going to waste on spa facials as I recently discovered is commonly being done. Instead, use raw local honey in limited amounts for beauty treatments, not this important medicinal honey!

Maple Syrup- The sugar maple tree offers the sap of its veins for us to use as food. Sap in its natural state is not terribly wonderful to eat, but cook it down and you have a wonderful sweet syrup. Keep in mind, this is one step removed from being natural. However, maple syrup is rich in beneficial minerals. So just a drizzle now and then of real, grade A maple syrup, and never, never, never pancake syrup which is not maple syrup at all!

Organic Unsulphured Blackstrap Molasses- High quality molasses is made from organic mature sugar cane and is a byproduct of refining the sugar. Organic sugar manufacturing does not involve using toxic chemicals compared to commercial molasses. The syrup remaining after the third boil has most of the sugar removed, does not taste sweet, and contains beneficial minerals, specifically calcium, magnesium, potassium, and iron. This is an important inclusion in all vegetarian diets or for those who avoid red meat. At most have a dose of one tablespoon daily on steel cut oats or in a healthy shake, but not as a baked goodie!

Sucanat- Pure, dried sugar cane juice is granular, dark brown, and unrefined. Sucanat contains everything the plant juice has to offer including the minerals that become part of molasses syrup. It still counts as sugar for calories, but is the most nutrient beneficial sugar. Only use sparingly as you would have used sugar or sugar substitutes.

Green Leaf Stevia- The sweetness of this plant is attributed to steviosides which are more concentrated in refined stevia versus green leaf. However, natural is always better, so green leaf stevia is the preference for both taste and quality. Stevia extract, a brown liquid also derived from the real plant, works well as a sweetener without the taste of a refined sweetener. The benefit is a no calorie, no carbohydrate sweet experience!

ARTIFICIAL SWEETENERS

"Open your eyes to the dangers of artificial sweeteners. The food industry wants you to eat artificial sweeteners because it is cheap not because they are better for you! Artificial sweeteners are no good for you and are usually in foods that aren't healthy for you anyway! SO STOP USING THEM!"—Dr. A

What the Bleep $#@! Can I Eat?

Aspartame- A.K.A. Nutrisweet, Equal, Spoonful- According to the Aspartame Consumer Safety Network, Aspartame is a direct nervous system irritant in part because it contains 50% phenylalanine which lowers the seizure threshold, blocks serotonin production leading to depression, contains aspartic acid which caused brain damage in animal testing, and methanol that damages liver and eyes. Aspartame also contains diketopiperazine which causes brain tumors in animal studies which caused it to fail FDA approval until a different politician came along and approved it despite the problems associated with its use. Aspartame has been associated with triggering symptoms of Alzheimers, epilepsy, Parkinsons, Multiple sclerosis, fibromyalgia, Graves disease, arthritis, brain tumors (astrocytoma, glioblastoma) and multiple organ related diseases.[xxv] Once Aspartame enters the human body, it heats up beyond 86 degree Farenheit and coverts to formaldehyde. Formaldehyde is a listen toxin used to preserve dead bodies! The patent no longer exists on Aspartame which means you have to read the ingredients on your product to see if aspartame is included.

Sucralose- A.K.A. Splenda- Sucralose was invented by scientists that were developing new pesticides and actually resembles the pesticide chemical DDT.[xxvi] Sucralose is not an innocent sugar substitute! Chemicals used to synthesize sucralose do not have to be listed on the label and in their own right are harmful including Acetone, Acetic acid, Acetyl alcohol, Acetic anhydride, Ammonium chloride, Benzene, Chlorinated sulfates, Ethyl alcohol, Isobutyl ketones, Formaldehyde, Hydrogen chloride, Lithium chloride, Methanol, Sodium methoxide, Sulfuryl chloride, Trityl chloride, Toluene, Thionyl chloride. According to a study in 2008, Splenda reduces the amount of good bacteria in the intestines by 50%, increases the pH level in the intestines, contributes to increases in body weight and affects the P-glycoprotein (P-gp) in the body in rejecting crucial health-related drugs being taken. The study researchers noted that the P-gp effect "could result in crucial medications used in chemotherapy for cancer patients, AIDS treatment and drugs for heart conditions being shunted back into the intestines rather than being absorbed by the body as intended."[xxvii]

Alcohol Sugars- sorbitol, mannitol, xylitol, erithrotol, isomalt, lactitol, maltitol, hydrogenated starch hydrolysates- do contain some calories, but do cause diarrhea, abdominal cramps and digestive problems which can occur at even low doses. Erithrotol causes the least amount of digestive side effects because it is more absorbable than the other alcohol sugars. There has been associated weight gain and elevated blood sugar associated with significant ingestion of alcohol sugars.[xxviii]

QUESTIONABLE SWEETENERS

Agave Nectar- Agave is really chemically refined hydrolyzed high-fructose inulin syrup and not raw or healthy as is claimed. True Agave nectar is fermented to make tequila, fermentation requires enzyme action, and the enzymes have to be destroyed in order to bottle the syrup. Most Agave syrup is imported from Mexico and there is a lot of speculation that corn syrup is added to keep their profits high.

JOHN KOHLER: AGAVE SYRUP: "THE TRUTH ABOUT AGAVE SYRUP, NOT AS HEALTHY AS YOU MAY THINK"[xxix]

. . . "Agave Syrup is advertised as "low glycemic" and marketed towards diabetics. It is true, that agave itself is low glycemic. We have to consider why agave syrup is "low glycemic." It is due to the unusually high concentration of fructose (90%) compared to the small amount of glucose (10%). Nowhere in nature does this ratio of fructose to glucose occur naturally. One of the next closest foods that contain almost this concentration of glucose to fructose is high fructose corn syrup used in making soda(HFCS 55), which only contains 55% fructose. Even though fructose is low on the glycemic index, there are numerous problems associated with the consumption of fructose in such high concentrations as found in concentrated sweeteners. . .

High Fructose Corn Syrup- this is a highly manufactured syrup that is nothing even close to natural. This inexpensive food sweetener is now being associated with increased risk of obesity, metabolic syndrome, and fatty liver, basically everything listed above regarding the agave syrup debate. Foods that used to say "natural" can no longer be labeled as such if they contain this ingredient because there's nothing natural about it!

Fructose- crystalline fructose powder tastes sweet like sugar, and is derived from cornstarch, Jerusalem artichoke, or dahlia bulbs, not from natural fruit. While it is touted as low glycemic and suitable for diabetics, it carries some risks associated with it. The most commonly reported problems are gas, bloating and diarrhea. Overconsumption leads to gout, non-alcoholic liver disease, increased appetite and overeating, elevated cholesterol and triglycerides, insulin resistance and obesity.[xxx]

Brown Rice Syrup- is manufactured from brown rice and barley sprout enzymes. Brown rice syrup is highly glycemic, even more so than ordinary table sugar so it is best to be avoided.

LOW GLYCEMIC RECIPES
Oat Protein Bars

- 2 cups Organic rolled oats
- ½ cup Quinoa, cooked, cooled
- ¼ cup Ground flax seeds

- ¾ cup Rice Protein Powder
- 1 tsp Baking soda
- ½ tsp Celtic Sea Salt
- ½ cup Chopped walnuts
- ½ cup Raw sunflower seeds
- ½ cup dried cranberries
- ½ cup Raw unsweetened coconut
- ½ cup Sucanat
- ½ cup Organic whole wheat flour
- ¼ cup Sunflower oil
- 2 tsp Frontier Organic Vanilla extract
- 1 cup Water

Place dry ingredients in a bowl, mix wet ingredients in a separate bowl before adding both together. Spread and press into oiled glass 9 x 13 pan. Bake at 350 for 20 minutes, cool, cut into squares.

Whole Grain Pilaf

¼ cup brown basmati rice
¼ cup quinoa
¼ cup steel cut oats
¼ cup amaranth
1 cup Pacific vegetable broth
1 cup pure water
¼ cup chopped nuts, lightly toasted in toaster oven
¼ cup dried currants
¼ tsp dried coriander
¼ tsp dried marjoram
Bring water and broth to boil, add grains, lower pot to simmer. After 20 minutes, add nuts, currants and herbs. Cook for another 10-15 minutes until grains are tender and water is absorbed into the grain.

Loaded Sweet Potato

Sweet potato or yam, one per person, baked, one per luncheon plate

Top with ½ teaspoon of coconut oil, 2 T. chopped pecans.
Sprinkle with 1 tsp ground flax seeds
Drizzle with a little Organic black strap molasses and pure maple syrup.
Sprinkle with Frontier Organics Pumpkin Pie Spice Blend and a little Celtic Sea salt.

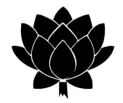

Chapter 6:
High Fiber Diet

Whatever you already know about fiber probably isn't what I am about to recommend! Many of my patients think they are eating a high fiber diet referring to their salads, fiber drinks, high fiber cereal and fiber bars. Salad vegetables are the lowest fiber vegetables, fiber drinks are not intended for daily use and shouldn't be needed in order to go to the bathroom, and the fiber in manufactured foods is indigestible, irritating and incomplete. Sorry to be the bearer of bad news!

Fiber-rich diets are indicated for those with constipation, diarrhea, irritable bowel, diverticulum, hormone imbalances, elevated cholesterol, intestinal bacterial imbalances, candida overgrowth, hormone imbalances, and for anyone trying to lower their risk of colon cancer, breast cancer, gallbladder disease, food allergies, immune problems and more. Generally the recommended amount of fiber is 25-35 grams daily as a combination of soluble and insoluble fiber spread out evenly at each meal.

Soluble fiber is the gooey fiber naturally found in foods. This is what makes the bowel movement bulky, feeds good bacteria that in turn makes nutrients to produce healthy cells in the intestinal tract.

Insoluble fiber is the "rough" fiber naturally found in foods. This is what makes the bowel movement move through at the proper rate. The roughness of insoluble fiber scrapes the bowel walls of any residue and cannot be digested by our system as it passes through. Together these fibers create good bowel health, regular bowel movements, and help eliminate cholesterol, hormones, and medications that need to be excreted.

For those of you with inflammatory bowel disease [ulcerative colitis, Crohn's] or irritable bowel disease, a high fiber diet can be aggravating to your bowel condition. For these conditions, soluble fiber is better tolerated than the insoluble fiber and highly manufactured fiber food products are completely out of the question. Steamed and lightly cooked fruits and vegetables are better tolerated than raw, and nuts or seeds are best taken as a butter form. Soluble pectin fiber powders are a good idea to include along with a digestive enzyme and probiotic supplements.

Refined foods have had their beneficial fiber removed. Manufactured foods that are "high in fiber" go to the trouble of adding the fiber back in, but typically it is in the form of insoluble fiber. Too much insoluble fiber intake leads to gas, cramps, diarrhea and aggravation of bowel inflammation due to the scraping, indigestible nature of this fiber.

I don't expect you to sit around calculating grams of fiber any more than you need to count grams of anything. Common sense and practicality needs to apply to all of your food selection. Whole grains, beans, berries, whole fruit with the peel, some vegetables, nuts and seeds all contain variable amounts of soluble and insoluble fiber. In the end, variety of texture and forms of foods will provide you with the proper balance.

The following table contains the foods with the highest amount of fiber in their edible state. Fiber charts can conflict with one another because of the difficulty and complexity of measuring this element of food. In general, all foods will have lower fiber content once they are cooked. I have taken into account that you wouldn't be eating an acorn squash raw, so the cooked fiber content is provided. Any fruit or vegetable that can be eaten raw has a raw fiber value listed.

Beneficial natural fiber is found in good amounts in the following foods:

Fiber Foods	Grams per 100g
Flax seeds	28
Amaranth	15.2
Bulgur wheat	9.0/cup
Elderberry	7.0
Macadamia nut	5.28
Peanuts, raw	4.85
Walnuts	4.60
Coconut, raw	4.27
Sunflower seeds	4.16
Blackberries	4.1
Apple	4.0
Guava	2.8-5.5
Pomegranate	3.4-5.0
Hazelnut, filbert	3.80
Dates	2.6-4.5
Raspberries	3.0
Corn, raw	2.90
Lentils	2.76
Almonds	2.71

Quinoa	2.6
Snow pea pod	2.50
Chickpeas	2.50
Currants	2.4
Black eyed peas	2.31
Brazil nut	2.29
Pumpkin seeds	2.22
Black beans	2.03
Adzuki bean	2.02
Avocado	2.11
Parsnip	2.0
Acorn squash	1.96
Brussels Sprouts	1.51
Leek	1.51
Kale/cabbage	1.50
Pear	1.4
Spaghetti squash	1.4
Celery root	1.30
Butternut squash	1.26
Artichoke	1.17
Broccoli	1.11
Green beans	1.10
Carrot	1.04
Escarole	0.90

Lettuce virtually has no fiber content, so don't think your salad is saving your health! Nuts and seeds with high fiber content can be sprinkled onto salad in small amounts packing a high fiber punch! Keep in mind that all grains are rather low in fiber once they are cooked and need to be introduced in limited amounts to make room for important foods like beans, berries and other foods listed above.

HIGH FIBER MEAL OPTIONS

"It's a challenge to eat 25 grams of fiber a day, but it can be done well with a little planning ahead!" –Dr. A

What is even more challenging is eating out at restaurants because whole grains and beans are scarce on the menu. Limit your restaurant dining if you are currently depending upon prescription or over-the-counter medicine to control diarrhea or constipation. Instead, adopt a fiber balanced diet and within two to three weeks you should notice a significant improvement.

Breakfast #1
¼ -½ cup blackberries
½ cup cooked plain steel-cut oats
2 tablespoons walnuts
1 tablespoon ground flax seeds

Breakfast #2
½ cup raspberries
½ cup fat-free Greek yogurt
¼ cup Ezekiel granola or Bob's Red Mill Muesli
1 teaspoon ground flax seeds

Lunch #1
1 cup lentil soup
WASA whole grain cracker
2 cups dark leafy greens for a salad
2 tablespoon pumpkin seeds as a salad topping
Handful pomegranate seeds [when available]
3 egg whites/3 oz chicken, turkey, fish, tofu
EVOO & lemon juice

Lunch #2

2 cups baby spinach as a salad base

½ cup black beans as a salad topping

2 tablespoons raw corn as a salad topping or added to salsa

Red pepper & Red onion

1 Tablespoons organic salsa

1 Tablespoons wholly guacamole

3 oz. tofu/chicken

Whole grain pita pocket- fill first with guacamole, then chicken/tofu, top with salsa

Snack #1

Handful snow peas/green beans

Baby carrots/red pepper

Hummus (chickpeas, tahini, lemon juice, cayenne, sea salt)

Snack #2

Grannysmith apple

2 tablespoons almonds or almond butter

Dinner #1

½ cup white beans

1 cup escarole

3 oz fish

1 cup cooked squash- zucchini, yellow

Dinner #2

½ cup broccoli

½ cup carrots

1 cup bok choy

½ cup mung bean sprouts

3 oz. chicken/fish/tofu

½ cup long cook brown rice

1 tablespoon sesame seeds

Dessert #1

½ cup pureed guava

1 teaspoon ground flax seeds

Lime juice

Raw honey

Chopped macadamia nuts

Dessert #2

Shredded raw coconut

Mango, diced

Cut wedges of pink grapefruit

Drizzle raw honey and sprinkle of cardamom

HIGH FIBER RECIPES

Cold Tabouleh Salad

2 cups cooked Bulgur wheat or quinoa prepared as directed

1 medium cucumber diced

1 medium tomato diced

½-1 cup chopped mint, cilantro and/or parsley

Olive oil, lemon juice, Celtic sea salt and pepper to taste

Serving Suggestions: Serve over a spinach salad with human and whole grain pita cut into wedges. Serve with Three Bean salad over lettuce greens. Serve with Curried Vegetables.

Three Bean Salad

1 can organic kidney beans, rinsed, drained

1 can organic garbanzo beans, rinsed, drained

[or use Eden Foods Salad Beans]
2 cups organic green beans cooked or frozen, thawed
EVOO, red wine vinegar, Celtic sea salt and pepper to taste

Black Eyed Pea Salad

1 can black eyed peas, rinsed and drained
4 pieces Applegate turkey bacon, cooked, cooled cut into crumbles
2-4 T. red onion, minced
1 mango, diced
1 red pepper diced
2 T. jalepeno, minced
EVOO, Apple cider vinegar, Celtic sea salt and cayenne pepper to taste

Shredded Slaw

1 cup shredded carrots
1 cup shredded red cabbage
1 cup shredded grannysmith apple
½ cup olive oil, ¼ cup organic apple cider vinegar warmed to melt 2 T.
honey, Celtic sea salt, cayenne pepper to taste
2 T. toasted sesame seeds [lightly toast them on a tray in the oven or
toaster oven]   Sprinkle with 2 T. ground raw chia or flax seeds.

Black Bean Chutney

1 can black beans, rinsed and drained
1 red bell pepper, diced
1-2 T. jalepeno pepper, minced
1-2 medium bodied fruit diced- mango, peach, nectarine, apricot
1 medium tomato, diced
1 medium onion, minced
Handful cilantro, minced
Juice of one lemon
EVOO, Celtic Sea Salt and cayenne pepper to taste

Serving Suggestions: Use on top of polenta, tofu, or fish. Serve with whole grain crackers and guacamole. Add to wraps for the filling.

Turkey Chili
1 lb. ground turkey
1 medium onion
1 red bell pepper & 1 green bell pepper
1 can light kidney beans, rinsed and drained
1 can dark kidney beans, rinsed and drained
1 can pinto beans, rinsed and drained
1 can fire roasted tomatoes
Chili powder (generous) and Celtic Sea Salt
Sauté turkey, onions and peppers in a little olive oil over medium heat until lightly browned, add rest of ingredients and cook over low heat until turkey cooked through, approximately 20 minutes.

HIGH FIBER POWDER SUPPLEMENTS

For those of you afraid to go without fiber powder, or who simply cannot or will not eat enough fiber, then including a fiber powder may be helpful. Keep in mind, not all fiber powders are created equal!

- Pectins- these are soluble fibers that are usually a clear or cloudy liquid when mixed with water providing bulk to the stool to hold more moisture and prevent constipation.
- Brans- these are insoluble fiber that are thick and usually mixed into food or drink producing a more rapid emptying of the bowel. Brans are also not truly a whole food and are missing the rest of the beneficial grain. Brans are not well suited to those with irritable bowel or inflammatory bowel disease.
- Seeds- flax and chia seeds are the most popular of these powders. They must be taken care of by refrigerating to prevent spoiling/rancidity and provide a combination of

soluble and insoluble fibers. Sometimes these produce gas and bloating that is undesirable which can be avoided by introducing just a teaspoon a day and working up to a tablespoon a day in the diet. Seeds are not well suited for those with diverticulum and active inflammatory bowel disease.

- Cleansers- these fiber blends often contain herbal medicines and/or clay binders that function as laxatives or stimulants as part of a colon cleanse and are not suitable for daily use. Chronic laxative abuse contributes to sluggish bowels when the stimulus is avoided. The best use of these powders is during an intentional cleansing program for a limited amount of time to assist with toxin removal.

Please note that I did not mention any commercially prepared fiber products, laxatives, or prescription liquids. I find these products to be completely unnecessary in most cases of digestive problems that I treat and the side effects unnecessary. Always looks to food first, then pectins, seeds and brans, and lastly for a fiber blend supplement.

Remember, this effort isn't just to have a bowel movement, this is about restoring normal health of the entire digestive tract that impacts on more than just the discomfort of your belly full of waste!

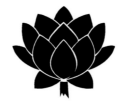

Chapter 7:
Antioxidant-Rich Diet

When you look in the mirror and see your body aging, the wrinkles and sagging is evidence of oxidative stress occurring inside of you. It's what you can't see that should worry you, not the worry lines! All day long our body makes free radicals that damage the DNA in our tissue creating what is referred to as 'oxidative stress.' On the outside it can look like moles, brown patches, gray hair, and wrinkles. On the inside it can look like inflammation and tissue damage. Antioxidants are believed to fight free radicals before they can create this damage thereby reducing the likelihood of diseased tissue and aging.

Our bodies produce antioxidant enzymes such as catalase, superoxide dismutase (SOD) and glutathione peroxidase that destroy free radicals with the help of manganese, zinc, copper and selenium for them to work properly. We need a steady stream of these nutrients and enzymes since free radicals are being formed all the time. Our body also produces an antioxidant, Coenzyme Q10, in our muscle as long as we have adequate B vitamins and vitamin C to help produce it. Combined with proper sleep habits and a healthy diet, we can slow down the process of aging.

Besides aging, conditions such as cataracts, macular degeneration, vascular disease, periodontal disease, cancer, heart disease, Alzheimer's, and Parkinson's are only some of the conditions associated with excessive oxidative stress. Protecting yourself from environmental pollutants, hydrating with pure water, minimizing emotional stress, and undertaking a reasonable but not excessive exercise program are also important factors in reducing overall oxidative stress. Other factors such as alcohol, smoking, and regular use of aspirin all increase the body's requirement for dietary and supplemental antioxidants. Infections are more likely to occur in those with excessive oxidative stress and inadequate dietary antioxidants as well.

Your level of oxidative stress can be measured by using the Oxystress Test Kit by North American Pharmacal suitable for at home use on a monthly basis. This simple urine test allows you to visualize how much oxidative damage is going on inside your body while monitoring your progress as you adopt a healthier lifestyle and antioxidant-rich diet to balance oxidative stress and repair. This is a must have test for anyone with cataracts or degenerative nervous system conditions!

Adopting an antioxidant-rich diet squelches oxidative stress thereby preventing excessive tissue damage. Even dairy farmers understand the need for balancing oxidative stress and repair for cows to successfully birth a calf and for adequate milk production by making sure they receive an antioxidant-rich diet.

Dietary antioxidants come in many forms. The First group is vitamins and minerals, namely vitamins A, C, E, selenium and Coenzyme Q10. The second group is botanical antioxidants such as carotenoids, isoflavones, flavonoids, and proanthocyanadins mainly found in deeply pigmented fruits and vegetables.
To keep it simple, basically eat the colors of the rainbow in the course

of the day, and to get specific, eat foods high on the ORAC scale. ORAC, Oxygen Radical Absorbance Capacity, values are assigned to foods indicating their ability to function as an antioxidant. The values are helpful for selecting foods that have the best potential for preventing damage in the body. The higher the ORAC value of the food, the better the action! In general, most nuts, berries and spices win hands down as the richest sources of dietary antioxidants.

ORAC FOOD VALUE CHART[xxxi]

Cloves, ground	314,446
Cinnamon, ground	267,536
Tumeric, ground	159,277
Acai berry, freeze dried	102,700
Parsley, dried	74,349
Basil, dried	67,553
Dark chocolate, unsweetened	49,926
Curry, dried	48,504
Sage, fresh	32,004
Mustard, yellow ground	29,257
Ginger, ground	28,811
Thyme, fresh	27,426
Marjoram, fresh	27,297
Goji berry	25,300
Chili powder	23,636
Pecans	17,940
Paprika, dried	17,919
Tarragon, fresh	15,542
Ginger root, raw	14,840
Elderberry, raw	14,697
Oregano, raw	13,970
Walnuts	13,541

Hazelnuts	9645
Savory, fresh	9465
Artichokes, boiled	9416
Blueberries	6552
Prunes	6552
Plums, raw	6259
Blackberries	5347
Garlic, raw	5346
Cilantro, raw	5141
Cabernet red wine	5034
Raspberries	4882
Basil	4805
Almonds	4454
Apple, grannysmith	3898
Apple, gala	2828
Strawberries	3577
Red currants, raw	3387
Figs, raw	3383
Cherries, sweet raw	3365
Peanuts	3166
Raisins	3037
Pears, raw	2941
Dates, medjool	2387
Broccoli, boiled	2386
Broccoli, raw	1362
Pomegranate, juice	2341
Red cabbage, raw	2252
Sweet potato, baked	2115
Chives	2094
Cashews, raw	1948
Oranges, naval	1819

What the Bleep $#@! Can I Eat?

Peaches, raw	1814
Alfalfa sprouts	1520
Red potato, baked	1326
Spinach, raw	1260
Grapes, red	1260
Green tea, brewed	1253
Lettuce, romaine	963
Cauliflower, raw	829
Sweet red pepper	791
Olive Oil, EVOO	684
Carrots, raw	666

By selecting the foods from this chart, you are providing yourself with a medley of antioxidant-rich foods. Foods not listed here either do not have an ORAC value assigned, the ORAC value was assigned to the uncooked food that cannot be eaten in that form (i.e. uncooked dried beans), or they were too low to consider including in the chart.

For example, take a look at typical salad ingredients:
- Lettuce-963
- Tomato- 367
- Cucumber- 214
- Celery- 497
- Onion- 614

Now, if you just add a few things to this salad, not the least of which is EVOO, you can boost the antioxidant value significantly:
- Artichoke hearts (9416), basil (67,553), sundried tomatoes and sweet red pepper (791)
- Grannysmith apple (3898), walnuts (13,541) and raisins (3037)
- Pear (2941), pecans (17,941), and red raspberries (1482)
- Spinach (1260), strawberries (3577), fresh garlic (5346) and alfalfa sprouts (1520)

- When available, a sprinkling of pomegranate seeds, delightful!

ANTIOXIDANT-RICH RECIPES

Create dishes that have berries, nuts and spices added for an extra antioxidant punch to each meal. The berries can be fresh or frozen and nuts should be raw, soaked overnight in water and rained, not roasted or salted. Nuts can also be processed into nutmilks or butters as well. For spices, I use Frontier Organics dried herbs and spices or fresh herbs from the garden.

- **Curry Powder** is an antioxidant-rich blend of coriander, turmeric, mustard, cumin, fenugreek, paprika, cayenne, cardamom, nutmeg, cinnamon and cloves and should be included in your cuisine.
- **Chili Powder** is a rich blend of antioxidant power from red chilis, cumin, oregano, coriander, garlic, allspice and cloves.
- **Chinese Five Spice Powder-** cinnamon, fennel, cloves, star anise, white pepper.
- **Herbs of Italy-** oregano, thyme, basil, garlic, black pepper, tarragon, red bell pepper, chives.
- **Pumpkin Pie spice-** cinnamon, ginger, cloves, nutmeg.

Antioxidant Smoothie

1 cup pomegranate juice (not from concentrate, not sweetened with other juices, just the tart stuff!)
¼ cup blackberries
1 wedge lime with peel
1 Tablespoon black elderberry syrup (from the health food store)
¼ tsp grated fresh ginger root
Drizzle of honey if needed for added sweetness
1 cup ice
Blend and serve with mint as a garnish

Fruit & Nut Truffles

½ cup each of dried dates, raisins, currants, goji or acai berries (1/4 cup at most) soaked together in orange juice for 4-6 hours, pour off remaining juice and set aside

½ cup each of almond, walnuts, pecans, soaked in warm water for 4-6 hours, then drained.

Using food processor, put in the soaked fruit and nuts and begin processing, adding the reserved juice if necessary until a thick doughy paste is formed.

Roll into 1" balls and dust with unsweetened cocoa powder mixed with cinnamon and ground ginger to taste

Serve in little candy papers as an appetizer or dessert

Breakfast Hash

1-2 pounds baby red/purple potatoes, scrubbed, cubed

1 red bell pepper, diced

1 medium onion, diced

1 large gala apple, cored, diced

1 zucchini, diced

1-2 tablespoons bruised thyme leaves and rosemary needles

EVOO, Celtic Sea Salt, Cayenne pepper to taste

After coating all the vegetables with the oil and herbs, place on a cookie sheet and bake at 425-450° for 30 minutes or until potatoes are fork tender. Turn vegetables halfway through cooking time.

Roasted Herbed Sweet Potatoes

As many sweet potatoes as people you want to feed, scrubbed, cut into long Texas fries, with the peel and all!

Fresh sage and rosemary, minced 1 tablespoon each per potato used

EVOO, Celtic Sea Salt and black pepper to taste

Toss together, place on cookie sheet, bake at 425-450° for 30 minutes until fork tender

Chicken/Tofu Curry

1 whole chicken, baked, skin removed, deboned, cubed or 1 package of tofu, cubed

Red grapes cut in half, same amount as you have of chicken/tofu

1 cup walnuts, coarsely chopped

Small bunch celery, sliced

Small onion, diced

2 large Tablespoons Vegennaise mayo, grapeseed oil version [rich in Coenzyme Q10]

Curry powder, a heavy handed dose until it's all very yellow!

Celtic sea salt to taste, and a little extra dose of cayenne/black pepper

Antioxidant All-Purpose Marinade

½ cup organic, wheat free tamari

¼ cup cabernet red wine

¼ cup sesame oil

¼ cup EVOO

1" piece fresh ginger root, grated

2 cloves garlic, pressed

1 Tablespoon Maple Syrup

1 tsp organic Worcestershire sauce

Celtic sea salt, black pepper

Whisk ingredients together, marinate meat or tofu, grill or bake as desired

Antioxidant All-Purpose Salad Vinaigrette

1 cup EVOO

½ cup organic red wine vinegar

2 Tablespoons green tea

2 Tablespoons Pomegranate Juice

1 clove garlic, pressed

½ tsp fresh grated ginger
1 Tablespoon minced fresh onion
Dried herbs to taste: oregano, basil, marjoram
Celtic sea salt, black pepper, pinch cayenne to taste
Whisk together and use on a tossed salad, a three bean salad, or roasted vegetable salad.

DRINK YOUR ANTIOXIDANTS?

Drinking your antioxidants is another way to receive cellular protection. Green tea has been touted as the antioxidant tea of choice. Coffee actually wins out when it comes to the potential antioxidant power in the mug. CNN recently reiterated that coffee is a good source of antioxidants, reflecting on research from 2005 to the present. Not that coffee has more antixodants than berries, it is drank more often so it has become the main antioxidant that Americans actually partake in their diet. So, for convenience, we will explore the benefits of beverages, but understand this is still a weak antioxidant compared to fruits and vegetables!

Coffee

The main antioxidants in coffee are chlorogenic acids (CGA's),which belong to the antioxidant group polyphenols, having the potential to protect against cardiovascular disease and cancer. [xxxii] Coffee has been shown to exhibit the highest polyphenol content compared to its tea and cocoa counterparts having four times as many antioxidants as green tea. [xxxiii]

My concern with drinking coffee is this, it is loaded with pesticides and contaminants, therefore, you must buy organic! Secondly, what you put in your coffee that can counteract the beneficial protection that antioxidants have to offer. Refined sugar, animal fat (cream) and chemicals (artificial creamers) are known contributors to cancer, diabetes and poor health. So keep it clean and simple, and don't add the syrups and junk that make drinking coffee a problem! Newman's Organic coffee can be found in most every grocery store and at the drive thru of McDonalds so it's not hard to succeed on this one! Use Sucanat or Stevia to sweeten and Organic Half & Half or Fat-free organic milk to lighten if desired.

Cocoa

The only truly healthy hot chocolate is when it is made from scratch. I have not found one mix that passes the test of being 'healthy.' It's not hard to make but it takes longer than just microwaving a cup of water. So, if you want your antixodants from chocolate, you're going to need a pan and a stove!

- Dagoba Authentic Cocoa Powder for hot chocolate
- Green & Black Hot Chocolate Powder

In 2003, Science Daily reported on a study from Cornell University that hot cocoa is the healthier choice to drink compared to red wine.[xxxiv] They found that hot cocoa had two times stronger antioxidants than red wine, 2-3 times stronger than green tea, and 4-5 times stronger than black tea. They also pointed out that the antioxidants are more available from the hot version rather than cold chocolate milk.

Lastly, even though chocolate is high in antioxidants, commercial candy bars are not the way to get your antioxidants because of chemical alkalai processing, saturated fats, and the refined sugars they contain. However, an *occasional* piece of 70% organic dark chocolate candy is not completely out of the question! [same brands- dagoba and green&black].

Teas

According to Dr. Weisburger, a leading researcher on the benefits of tea, tea has 8 to 10 times the antioxidant power of fruits or vegetables. Dr. Weisburger also reports that they found green and black tea to have the same amount of polyphenols. The USDA lists thearubigins, epicatechins, and catechins as the flavonoid antioxidants tea contains. Preferentially, green and white teas are somewhat healthier because they are not fermented, but all tea has something good to offer. Again, I am recommending organic to avoid unnecessary pesticide exposure or fumigants that may be used on imported teas.

Chai

The ingredients in Chai are some of the highest on the antioxidant chart above. Premade Chai, however, is typically weaker than homemade and much more 'sugared up.' Take the time to make it from scratch and enjoy it hot or cold! These are also the same spices you will find in blends such as chili powder, pumpkin pie spices, curry powder, and Chinese five spice powder. So just add Chai to your list of good for you [from scratch] spicy food!

Making Chai Tea from Scratch

(directly sourced from Simply Recipes.com)

Spice ingredients for one pot of Chai tea:

1/2 of a star anise star

10-12 whole cloves

6-7 whole allspice

1 heaping teaspoon of cinnamon bark (or 2 short sticks)

6-7 whole white peppercorns

1 cardamon pod opened to the seeds

Other ingredients:

1 cup water

4-6 cups whole milk

2 heaping tablespoons of a high quality full-bodied broad-leaf black tea (Ceylon, or English Breakfast if a broad-leaf Ceylon is not available)

Sucanant/honey

In a 2-qt saucepan, add spices to 1 cup of water. Bring to a boil; remove from heat; let steep for 5-20 minutes, depending on how strong a spice flavor you want.

Add 4-6 cups of whole milk to the water and spices. If you don't have whole milk, you can also use non-fat or low-fat milk, just add some cream to it, a few tablespoons. Bring the milk and spice mixture just to a boil and remove from heat.

Add the tea to the milk and let steep for 5 to 10 minutes to taste. (Option at this point - reheat to a simmer and remove from heat.) You can add sugar at this point, or serve without sugar and let people put the amount of sugar in they want. Traditionally, sugar is added before serving. Strain into a pot. Serve. Add sugar to taste.

Wine

Grapes are loaded with antioxidants, so much so that the whole grape, including seeds, stems and leaves, are considered worthy of being used for medical purposes. So at the very least, eat dark grapes with seeds and actually eat some of the seeds! In general, the polyphenol antioxidants in red wine are believed to protect the lining of the blood vessels. Specifically, Resveratrol, a flavonoid antioxidant in red wine, is believed to prevent damage to blood vessels, reduce bad cholesterol, prevent blood clot formation and possibly reduce inflammation in the body. [xxxv]

Sangria

Add the benefits of citrus bioflavonoids to wine by making Sangria:

1 Bottle Organic Red Wine- Pino Noir, Cabernet
1 Lemon cut into wedges
1 Orange cut into wedges
2 Tablespoons honey
1-3 Tablespoons organic brandy flavoring
2 cups sparkling mineral water

ANTIOXIDANT SUPPLEMENTS

When oxidative stress is high on testing or by virtue of multiple stressors or diagnosis, then dietary sources of antioxidants is not enough. Obtaining antioxidants from a variety of sources is highly recommended.

Vitamin-Mineral Formula

A combination of vitamins A, C, E, and minerals zinc, selenium and manganese should be the very least of what a formula should contain. Cofactors such as B vitamins, reduced glutathione, and bioflavonoids are also helpful to enhance the antioxidant effect.

- *Metamorphosis Products Cell-Protect Antioxidants™* is a blend of naturally sourced vitamins A, C, E, the minerals selenium, manganese and cofactors round out this formula. Taken as one capsule daily as the beginning of protecting against cellular damage.

Botanical Formula

Plants are best used as extracts medicinally, rather than just dried plant material with nutrients that are still unavailable. Pine bark, red grape and green tea are at least the best sources of extracts to begin with.

- *Metamorphosis Products Tissue-Protect™* is a combination of Pycnogenol (pine bark extract), Resveratrol and Red Grape (seeds, skins, stems), Bilberry extract, Green tea extract, ginkgo extract (with reduced of headache producing ingredients, a common side effect of ginkgo), milk thistle extract and citrus bioflavonoids. The quality of these botanicals surpasses most on the market since this is not dried plant material, instead all the beneficial part of the plant was naturally extracted from the fiber of the plant. These extracts are contaminant free and full of the antioxidant medicine that the plants have to offer. Taken as one capsule twice daily is the next step towards producing healthy tissue such as eyes, blood vessels (including varicose veins and hemorrhoids), gums, and more.

Amino Acid Formula

There are certain amino acids, botanicals and cofactors that help protect liver and gastrointestinal tissue. Typically glutathione, milk thistle and alpha-lipoic acid get all the attention, but a full spectrum formula is often the better choice.

- *Metamorphosis Products Hepato-Protect™* is a combination formula of milk thistle extract, N-Acetyl-Cysteine, Alpha-Lipoic Acid, L-Methionine, L-Cysteine, Taurine, and Trimethylglycine. Taken as one capsule twice daily, it supports proper liver function assisting in the removal of toxins that contribute to oxidative stress, but also assists in protecting liver and gastrointestinal tissue.

Food Concentrates

There are a variety of powders and drinks on the market touting their high antioxidant value. The problem with some of these formulas is that the quality may be lacking. Powders are often dried plant material and not extracts, making the nutrients less available and less beneficial. Juices are often loaded with fruit juice concentrates that add sugar to your diet. There are even some drinks in fancy wine bottles with lots of marketing hype and two unwanted preservatives to boot!

Here are the food concentrates I tend to recommend because the quality is what it should be regarding plant extracts:

- *Jarrow, High Berry Powder*®
- *Garden of Life, Radical Fruits Antioxidant Complex*®
- *Biotics Research, Nitrogreens*®

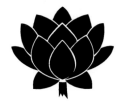

Chapter 8:
Omega-3 Balanced Diet

Omega-3 fatty acids are considered "essential" because the body cannot make them and they must be included in the diet in order for the body to remain healthy. Linoleic and alpha-linoleic acids must be included in the diet for other fatty acids to be assembled. Omega-3 oils are necessary for proper brain function such as memory, performance and behavior, and for normal growth and development. These special oils possess anti-inflammatory action being shown to be effective against heart disease, arthritis and cancer among many other conditions that involve inflammation.

I'm here to remind you that not all fat is necessarily bad. Some fat in your diet is necessary for good health and is required for many basic body processes. Children and pregnant women especially need adequate fat for healthy development of their nervous system and for proper growth and development.

Benefits of fats:

- Efficiently provide calories for energy
- Required to support cell growth

- Help protect the body's organs and keep the body warm
- Help the body absorb some nutrients (including vitamins A, D, E, and K)
- Needed for production of important hormones

Fish oil is one source of beneficial omega-3 fat. According to National Institutes of Health, "Fish oil contains docosahexaenoic acid (DHA) and eicosapentaenoic acid (EPA), while some nuts (English walnuts) and vegetable oils (canola, soybean, flaxseed/linseed, olive) contain alpha-linolenic acid (ALA). Fish or fish oil supplements lowers triglycerides, reduces the risk of death, heart attack, dangerous abnormal heart rhythms, and strokes in people with known cardiovascular disease, slows the build-up of atherosclerotic plaques ("hardening of the arteries"), and slightly lowers blood pressure."[xxxvi]

The standard American diet, referred to as "S.A.D" for what it represents nutritionally, delivers more omega-6 fatty than omega-3 fatty acids. Omega-6 fatty acids promote inflammation causing damage to tissue. Dietary intake should provide more omega-3 than omega-6 to keep inflammation in control. Eating refined carbohydrates and sugars signals the body to produce additional omega- 6, an inflammatory trigger in the body.

Signs and symptoms of inadequate of omega-3 intake includes at the very least fatigue, poor memory, dry skin, heart problems, high cholesterol, mood swings or depression, and poor circulation. The overall nutrition goal is to increase omega-3 intake and minimize but not completely eliminate omega-6. Vegetarians often need to look for ways to keep omega-6 fatty acids in their diets to keep themselves in balance as well, such as including sunflower and safflower oil in their diets.

National Institutes of Health recommends people should consume at least 2% of their total daily calories as omega-3 fats. To meet this recommendation, a person would have to eat at least 2 grams of omega-3 fats if consuming a 2000 calorie diet. Some experts believe that this recommendation is not high enough and recommend at least 4% of their total calories (approximately 4 grams) as omega-3 fats. According to the Dietary Guidelines for Americans (DGAs), dietary fat intake should be between 20 and 35 percent of the total daily calories. On a 2,000 calorie diet, 30 percent (mid-range)of calories from fat would equal 65g. In addition, the DGAs recommend that most fats come from sources of polyunsaturated and monounsaturated fatty acids, such as fish, nuts, seeds, olives, avocados and vegetable oils.

DHA is the most important aspect of omega-3 intake for pregnant women and developing babies [and for breast cancer prevention]. While there are no set daily intake requirements, it is generally agreed upon to provide 200-300 mg DHA daily to the mother for pregnancy and lactation to benefit the neurological growth and development of the baby. Many fish are also a source of environmental contaminants and are not recommended for pregnant and lactating women, making supplementation a necessity. Not all fish oil products are high in DHA unless they are specifically formulated for pregnancy, and many are not screened for contaminants [see omega-3 supplementation section].

OMEGA 3 FOOD CHOICES[xxxvii]
Select from the chart below for foods and spices high in omega-3 to include in your everyday meals. Values of are per 100 gram serving for equal comparison.

Flax seeds	8543 mg
Chia seeds	7164 mg
Fish caviar	5388 mg

Fish roe	3405 mg
Radish seed sprouts	3358 mg
Salmon, wild atlantic raw	2843 mg
Walnuts	2276 mg
Basil	2747 mg
Oregano	2732 mg
Cloves	2649 mg
Mackeral, atlantic raw	2605 mg
Grape leaves	2443 mg
Marjoram	2384 mg
Anchovy, raw	2257 mg
Herring, raw	2188 mg
Spinach, frozen	2183 mg
Tarragon	2004 mg
Oysters, raw	1977 mg
Spearmint	1959 mg
Capers, canned	1600 mg
Striped bass, raw	1586 mg
Rainbow trout, raw	1567 mg
Alfalfa seeds sprouts	1522 mg
Mustard, prepared yellow	1457 mg
Cauliflower	1452 mg
Sardines, canned	1423 mg
Sea bass, raw	1382 mg
Arugala	1360 mg
Romaine lettuce	1329 mg
Peppermint	1243 mg
Halibut	1181 mg
Lamb	1179 mg

There are many more foods with omega-3, too many to mention, but it is more important to understand the categories of foods that are naturally high in omega 3- nuts, greens, herbs, spices, and fish.

Easy Omega 3 Choices- Grams per Serving[xxxviii]
- Flax seeds (unheated) ¼ cup serving (7 g)- usually eaten as 1-3 teaspoons per day as a serving.
- Walnuts (unheated) ¼ cup serving (2.3 g)
- Navy beans, kidney beans 1 cup serving (0.2-1.0 g)
- Tofu 4 oz. serving (0.4 g)
- Fish (not fried) 4 oz serving- salmon (2 g), scallops (1.1 g), halibut (0.6 g), shrimp (0.4 g), snapper (0.4 g), tuna (0.3 g)
- Winter squash 1 cup serving (0.3 g)
- Olive oil (unheated) 1 oz. (0.2 g)

PRIMER ON GOOD VS. BAD FAT

You will never hear me tell a patient that fat is to be avoided. In fact I make sure it is budgeted into everyone's diets to provide an array of benefits that only plant fat can provide. There are even patients who need to eat egg yolks to re-establish normal hormone function in their body. What they do with that yolk, that's the problem. Most of the beneficial oils must be protected from heat, light, and air to prevent oxidation [a.k.a. rancidity]. Rancid oils contribute to the inflammatory response in the body making them an undesirable inclusion in the diet. Plant fats will never cause as much trouble as animal fat unless they are mishandled.

Saturated Fat [butter, coconut oil]- There is no hard evidence that saturated fat, more specifically coconut oil, causes damage in the human body. What is true, however, is that animal fat containing arachidonic acid and high intake of omega-6 oils creates inflammation in the body. Inflammation is the enemy, not coconut oil! The American Heart Association recommends limiting saturated fats to less than 7% of your daily intake, basically 16 grams per 2000 calorie diet.

Coconut oil is one of the most heat tolerant oils and is resistant to rancidity. Coconut oil also supports proper thyroid function and is especially helpful when taken with fruit. Coconut contains lauric acid, possessing antiviral activity, and caprylic acid having antifungal activity, both helpful for immune related issues as well. Coconut oil is also rich in medium-chain triglycerides that are shown to improve athletic performance, lower blood sugar, regulate appetite, only minimally contributes to body fat compared to other fats, are used to repair tissue damage, and fuels the brain for improved cognitive function. **COCONUT OIL, NOT AS BAD AS YOU THINK!**

Polyunsaturated Fat [corn, safflower, sunflower, sesame, soy oils]- All polyunsaturated oils are susceptible to rapidly oxidizing from heat, light or air causing free radical damage in the body. Polyunsaturated oils have been linked with cancer development, specifically breast,[xxxix] and contributes to cancer metastasis overall.[xl] Even though a food may deliver polyunsaturated fats, many contain monounsaturated fats as well, see the table below for the best monounsaturated fat choices. **HEATED POLYUNSATURATED FATS, BAD!**

Monounsaturated fat [olive oil, avocado]- The foods high in this fat still have some polyunsaturated or saturated fat, but mostly contain oleic acid believed to be highly beneficial. One report on olive oil and atherosclerosis reveals that particles of LDL cholesterol ("bad cholesterol") that contain the monounsaturated fats of olive oil are less likely to become oxidized. Oxidized cholesterol builds thick artery walls by forming plaque that can cause a heart attack or stroke.[xli] A recent study from researchers at Universitat Autònoma de Barcelona, led by Dr Eduard Escrich, have discovered a key mechanism by which virgin olive oil, in contrast to other vegetable oils, protects the body against breast cancer.[xlii] Basically, Olive oil was found to put breast cancer into reverse, whereas, corn oil steps on the accelerator for breast tumor growth. Now, more than ever before, we need the highest quality olive oil to be part of the daily diet in adequate amounts. **OLIVE OIL, ALL GOOD, GOOD, GOOD!**

Per 100 grams serving[xliii]	Monounsaturated Fat Grams
Sunflower oil, high oleic	83 g
Safflower oil	74g
Olive oil	70g
Macadamia nuts, raw	58g
Hazelnuts	45g
Pecans, raw	40 g
Almonds, raw	32 g
Peanuts, Brazil nuts, Pistachios, raw	25g
Avocado, Haas, raw	9.8g

Cooking Oil Quality- Manufactured oils that are not organic or naturally pressed use chemicals such as benzene or hexane in the process of extracting the oil from the plant. [xliv] Since benzene is not allowed into the food supply, the oils have to be heated to burn off the benzene before bottling contributing to rancidity and the formation of trans-fats. Chemical anti-foaming agents are also added to cooking oils for high heat use. Commercial spray cooking oils contain propellants along with additives making it no longer natural or helpful for your overall health. High quality oils have not been extracted with chemicals, are protected from heat, light and air, and are often bottled in amber or green glass to protect it from light once bottled. Use the Misto sprayer with your own organic high quality oil if you want to spray oil on foods or into pans.

Always choose organic, cold expeller pressed, unrefined oils for eating. First press has the highest level of antioxidants—Dr. A

Spreads and Butters
All margarines as produced by hydrogenating oil, creating trans-fats and often contain soy oil or canola oil that are easily oxidized. The only margarine that seems to have gotten it right is "Earth Balance" because it is high in omega-3, has no trans-fats, and no soy or canola oil. It does, however, contain some defatted soybean for those who are allergic or are concerned about the possible hormone effect. Don't kid yourself thinking that butter is necessarily better. Cream is loaded with animal hormones and arachidonic acid (a.k.a. inflammation) whether they received medicinal hormones or not. Olive oil on foods or the use of nut butters, avocado, or tahini/hummus are your best choices to increase your good fat intake via spreads or bread.

Nut butters are available from peanuts, almonds, cashews, macadamias, hazelnuts, sunflower seeds, pumpkin seeds, and sesame seeds (a.k.a. tahini). Most every question you could have about the quality of nut butters can be answered by www.worldpantry.com who manufacture Maranatha nut butters. Nuts and seeds are a great source of beneficial omega fatty acids and monounsaturated oils.
Deep Fried Foods- Heat oxidizes oils and creates free radical damage in the body. Deep fried foods are cooked in oils that have become rancid from high heat and repeated use and contain acrylamides from potatoes and bread coatings that were fried in the oil. Unfortunately, potato and tortilla chips fall into this category as well. The International Agency for Research on Cancer considers acrylamides a "probable human carcinogen," based on studies in laboratory animals.[xlv] You would need to consume a large amount of antioxidants to remedy the ill effects of this much oxidative damage from fried

foods. Every year at Thanksgiving I think of all the people deep frying their turkeys in peanut oil, it's an abomination of how to properly cook food! Even though peanut oil is preferred for frying because it does not form trans fats with high heat, a 1998 study from Wistar Institute in Philadelphia showed that peanut oil contains a compound called lectin that causes increased plaque buildup on artery walls.[xlvi] **DEEP FRIED FOODS, BAD!**

Trans-Fat- The Mayo Clinic reports that trans-fats raise LDL "bad cholesterol" and lowers HDL "good cholesterol." Trans-fats are not found in nature, they are manufactured by hydrogenating oils. "Partially hydrogenated" or "shortening" on the ingredient list is your clue that the food item contains trans fats. [xlvii] Margarines, peanut butters, anything thick and gooey are suspect of having trans-fats, and many processed and packaged foods contain trans fats. **TRANS-FATS, BAD (even the USDA agrees with me)!**

Fake Fat [olestra, canola oil]- O.K. this is where I go absolutely nuts about what is allowed in our food supply!!! Olestra is a manufactured fat substitute sold under the name of Olean from Proctor and Gamble, a company known for manufacturing EVERYTHING BUT FOOD! Manufactured food products such as chips and baked goods containing olestra used to carry a warning label. Not any more according to the Center for Science in the Public Interest, **"In August 2003 the FDA dropped its requirement for a warning label on packages of olestra-containing chips. The label had read, "This product contains Olestra. Olestra may cause abdominal cramping and loose stools. Olestra inhibits the absorption of some vitamins and other nutrients. Vitamins A, D, E and K have been added."**

Olestra has also been associated with malabsorption of carotenoids, a major group of antioxidants.[xlviii] As it is, it's hard enough to get enough of the right form of vitamin D or K into people to protect bones and breast tissue. Who exactly needs more ways to create oxidative damage in their body? Nobody!   In my opinion, olestra should never have been allowed into food. It doesn't matter if they add vitamins into this fat-free junk food, you need your own vitamins to stay put and keep you healthy! **F.Y.I.-DON'T DIET WITH JUNK FOOD FOR WEIGHT LOSS IN THE FIRST PLACE!!!!!**

Besides olestra, there is nothing natural or beneficial about canola oil either, at least from everything I have read! It doesn't matter if they [the Canadian government and The American Heart Association] say it's high in omega-3 and is monounsaturated, it has other problems that no one is talking about.

First, there is no such thing as a canola plant. Canola oil is manufactured from rape seed and given the name Canola which stands for 'Canadian Oil, Low Acid.' Originally used as a pesticide and an industrial lubricant, rape seed oil is from the mustard family and contains high amounts of toxic erucic acid associated with the formation of fibrotic heart damage.

A newer variety of rape seed plant was formed when the war industry died producing a plant with lower acid content making it more 'people friendly,' but some research still points to the risk of heart disease from the presence of erucic acid. Sally Fallon, author of Nourishing Traditions, notes that the omega–3 fatty acids of processed canola oil are transformed during the deodorizing process (because the smell is awful and inedible) into trans–fatty acids because of the high temperature (reportedly 300 degrees or more). Fallon reports one study indicating "heart healthy" canola oil actually created a deficiency of vitamin E, one of our main antioxidants necessary for heart health! Dr. Enig also writes extensively about how canola oil is loaded with trans-fats![xlix] Canola oil can also be high in sulphur making it more vulnerable to rancidity and another possible source of allergens in processed foods. Just what you need . . . more trans-fats, less antioxodants and more rancidity with oxidative damage making you sick and aged! Are you lining up to get some yet? **OLESTRA AND CANOLA, BAD, BAD, BAD [in my opinion, and I'm in good company]!**

FAT HEALTHY RECIPES

Breakfast Parfait

Using a parfait or goblet glass, place a spoonful of berries at the bottom, sprinkle in 1 T. chopped walnuts, a sprinkle of granola or muesli, sprinkle with ½ tsp ground flax seeds, and add a glob of organic Greek yogurt. Repeat these layers again. Top off with a drizzle of raw local honey and a sprinkle of cinnamon.

Salmon Salad

3 oz. piece of wild Alaskan salmon per person, steamed, cooled, flaked into bowl or canned, boned. Chopped onion, chopped celery, Vegennaise (enough to bring it together but not too gooey), Celtic sea salt and ground black pepper to taste, and a generous sprinkle of dill weed.

Herb & Vegetable Stuffed Fish

Any white fish filet, rinsed, patted dry
Smear the top side of the fish with organic mustard
Place a handful of soft herbs across the center of the filet- parsley, cilantro, dill or basil
Place thin cut spears of yellow squash, zucchini or tomato in the center
Place a thin slice of lemon on top
Roll up the fish over the herbs and vegetables and fix into place with a toothpick.
Place in glass dish, give them a drizzle of EVOO, bake at 350° for 30 minutes until fish is flakey.

<u>Alternative cooking method:</u> place all ingredients into a parchment paper pouch: cut a piece of parchment about 12" x 12", wet with water, place the fish and toppings in the center, fold up the paper and tuck the ends into place, baste the entire outside of the pouch with any vegetable oil, place on grill on medium-high for 30 minutes.

Tarragon Chicken
4 boneless, skinless chicken breasts rinsed, patted dry, cut into halves. Using any kind of flour, add salt and pepper to the flour and dredge each piece of chicken. Slowly heat 1 T. olive oil and 1 T. coconut oil in a skillet, lightly brown each side of the chicken over medium-low heat. Remove chicken from the pan and add the following ingredients to the pan: 1 onion sliced, 2 large carrots sliced, and cook until soft. Add one cup of organic chicken broth (Pacific) to the pan and ½ cup organic white wine, add the chicken back into the pan and simmer on low to completely cook the chicken. Take out the chicken and vegetables with a slotted spoon, add 2-4 oz. of Thai coconut milk, 1 T. Dijon mustard, 4 T. chopped fresh tarragon (or 2 T. dried), and 1 T. arrowroot, whisk together while simmering until thickened. Serve one piece of chicken with vegetables and a whole grain such as Quinoa and pour the sauce over the top. This recipe can also easily be made with fish or tofu instead of chicken. Enjoy!

All Purpose Basic Vinaigrette
½ cup Organic red wine or apple cider vinegar
1 cup First cold pressed EVOO
2 Tablespoons Pure water
½ Onion, chopped
1 clove Garlic, pressed
¼ tsp. Oregano, dried
¼ tsp. Marjoram, dried
¼ tsp. Basil, dried

¼ tsp. Celery seed, ground

¼ tsp. Coriander, ground

[I only recommend fresh herbs if you are using the whole batch and do not plan on storing it]

Celtic Sea Salt and ground Black Pepper to taste

Blend until well mixed. Refrigerate.

Healthy Pesto

This recipe is traditional pesto minus the grated cheese. I'm sure you'll find ways to get cheese in your diet anyhow, but try this on for size and see how you like it!

½ cup First cold pressed EVOO

¼ cup Pine nuts

¼ cup Walnuts

2 cups Fresh Basil

3 cloves garlic, pressed/minced

Celtic sea salt and ground black pepper to taste.

Put the nuts and basil into a food processor and pulse to break down. Add the garlic. While processing, slowly add the olive oil until all ingredients are mixed well and slightly coarse. Season to taste. Toss onto steamed vegetables, greens, tofu, chicken, fish, whole grain pasta, etc. Freeze pesto in ice cube trays for an easy way to keep this in your diet through the winter. Of course this insinuates that it summertime and you are growing the basil and care about it being fresh and organic, otherwise you can make pesto all year round from basil at the grocer!

Mediterranean Picnic/Party Platter

Organic roasted red pepper hummus

Baba ganoush

Mediterranean Organic brand stuffed grape leaves

Mediterranean Organic whole green olives with lemon

Mediterranean Organic whole mixed party olives
Artichoke hearts packed in water or oil
Steamed Asparagus tossed in olive oil and lemon juice
Ezekiel brand pita pockets (or GFL Foods gluten-free pita), cut into wedges
Cover a large platter with greens- arugala and/or baby spinach. Use ramekin dishes for the hummus and baba ganoush and place on the platter. Arrange the rest of the ingredients attractively on the platter. For added color, include organic baby carrots and long slices of organic roasted red peppers. Serve next to the basket of pita wedges. I also serve tabouleh and cucumber raita with this: diced cucumber tossed in plain yogurt, seasoned with dill and Celtic sea salt. Yum!!!

Fresh Guacamole
1-2 medium Haas avocados that easily dent when squeezed, mash with fork
1 medium tomato chopped
1-2 T. cilantro finely chopped
1-2 T. fresh lemon juice
Cayenne pepper and Celtic Sea Salt to taste
Mix together with fork, place the pit into the bottom of the bowl to prevent browning. Serve with fresh cut vegetables.

Dr. A's Ceviche
If I hadn't been to Baja Mexico for missionary work, I would never have known how outstanding authentic Ceviche is! This version uses cooked instead of raw fish, but tastes divine nonetheless! Vegetarians can use firm tofu in place of the seafood and add a little seaweed to the recipe for the same great result.
Per person ingredients:
1-2 Sea scallops, rinsed, steamed until cooked through
1-2 large shrimp, rinsed, deveined, shelled, boiled until cooked through

1-2 oz white fish fillet, steamed until cooked through
Batch ingredients (remember, I don't measure!):
Ripe tomatoes, chopped
Onion, chopped
Cilantro, chopped
Fresh lemon and lime juice
Celtic Sea Salt, Cayenne pepper to taste
Coarsely chop the seafood into pieces, add to the rest of the ingredients, mash the ingredients with your clean bare hands to bring all the flavors together. Let it sit in a covered bowl on the top shelf of the fridge for 1-2 hours, serve in parfait or goblet glasses lined with mixed baby greens at the bottom. Garnish with a wedge of lemon and sprig of cilantro. Immediately Enjoy!

OMEGA 3 SUPPLEMENTATION

Prenatal Omega 3

Prenatal Omega 3 supplements need to provide between 200-300 mg DHA, be screened for contaminants such as mercury, cadmium, PCB's, dioxins, lead and other contaminants, and also be protected from oxidation [a.k.a. rancidity]. These supplements fulfill this criteria:

- *Jarrow Formulas® Preg-Natal® + DHA* functions as a great quality prenatal vitamin packet containing easily digested vitamins and minerals in their proper forms and amounts plus a capsule of omega oil providing 250 mg DHA. BY FAR THIS IS MY TOP PICK FOR WOMEN TO USE OVER ANY OTHER PRENATAL VITAMIN!
- *Metamorphosis Products Pristine HP O3™* provides 270 mg DHA per fish oil capsule.
- *Spectrum Prenatal DHA Softgels-* provides 200 mg of vegetarian algae sourced DHA in a vegetarian capsule.

Fish Oil Supplementation

As with prenatal vitamins, all fish oil supplements need to be screened for mercury, cadmium, PCB's, dioxins, lead and other contaminants. The oils need to be protected from rancidity the entire time they are handled and the encapsulation process should not involve benzene or hexane contamination. Third party testing should confirm the purity and stability of the final product to withstand oxidation and rancidity. Burping up fish oil is often a sign that the oil in the capsule is rancid. ALWAYS STORE YOUR FISH OIL CAPSULES IN THE REFRIGERATOR ONCE THEY ARE OPENED.

- Metamorphosis Products Pristine HPO3™ is a high potency fish oil capsule that delivers 360 mg of EPA and 270 mg of EPA per 1000 mg capsule making it 63% fish oil. Compare this to most commercial brands that deliver much less medicinal fish oil per 1000 mg capsule because of fillers.
- *Metamorphosis Products Pristine O3 Gems™* are smaller and well suited for use in children or adults who have difficulty swallowing larger capsules. Each 500 mg capsule provides 150 mg EPA and 100 mg DHA, taken as 1-6 capsules a day based on age and condition.
- *Metamorphosis Products Omega 3:6:9™* is a blend of fish, flax, borage and conjugated linoleic acid oils. This formula is well suited to those with a poor diet or are trying to lose weight.

Omega 3 Seed Supplementation

- *Ground Flax Seeds-* Ground flax seeds are an important source of lignans associated with the prevention of breast cancer. The extracted oil on the other hand is not as rich in lignans and is missing the beneficial fiber. Buy vaccuum packed foil bags of ground seeds, press out the air and zip seal, store in refrigerator to prevent oxidation. Use 1-3 teaspoons daily on food, press all the air out of the bag before sealing and refrigerate. Do not cook with flax seeds since heat destroys the beneficial omega 3 oils potentially causing liver problems.

- *Ground Chia Seeds*- contains 25-30% oil mostly in the form of alpha-linoleic (ALA). Treat the seeds the same as you do flax.

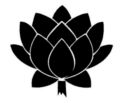

Chapter 9: O.S.F.A. Diet "One Size Fits All"

Everyone needs antioxidants, fiber and good plant fats to be healthy. This diet contains whole food meal suggestions that will accomplish more than any medication or supplement alone can do. You can literally stop disease in its tracks and sometimes even reverse damage just by correcting dietary indiscretions.

Are you ready?! There is no thinking involved at all in this chapter. Stock your kitchen, sharpen your knives, and hone your cooking skills to prepare any or all of these meals. There is nothing boring about the foods being recommended, but they are exactly the tastes that nature intended without the addictive flavors of artificial chemicals, salts, and manufactured sugars. If you have an allergen to any of the foods, simply eliminate and replace with a hypoallergenic alternative listed in the previous chapters. If you are vegetarian, use beans or tofu in place of the meat/fish/egg.

STOCKING THE PANTRY

Please assume everything is organic unless I say otherwise, it may not be available in organic form. I have purposefully not included certain items that are not the best form of an item, such as balsamic vinegar (carmelized syrup). So please assume that I intend for certain foods to be absent from the list rather than they have been forgotten. Also consider that these are the basics. Once we get into packaged foods, you have to read the ingredient lists to see what you can have.

Now get a box, and get rid of whatever is in your cabinet that is not on this list of good food, scrutinize it carefully based on everything you have learned, and only give it to your worst enemy if you just can't bring yourself to throw it away! Start with junk food and move on to the rest.

ORGANIC WHENEVER POSSIBLE!

Search for organic or natural as your first choices. Pantry items listed in **bold** are definitely to be included in your shopping for healthy foods to fill your cupboards.

Condiments: store in a lower cabinet away from heat, refrigerate the perishable goods, and refrigerate all items with an asterick* once the bottle is opened.

Apple cider vinegar
Red wine vinegar
Country Dijon mustard*
Ketchup*
Extra virgin, first cold pressed olive oil
Sunflower oil, high oleic (Spectrum)
Safflower oil, high oleic (Spectrum)
Virgin coconut oil
Lemon juice*
Vegennaise grapeseed mayo
Unpasteurized miso paste
Earth Balance spread [optional; not to use for cooking, just spreading]

What the Bleep $#@! Can I Eat?

Coconut milk, small cans
Tahini
Hummus
Wholly guacamole
Salsa*
Bragg Organic Healthy Vinaigrette
Pacific brand 4-pack vegetable broth*
Nut butters*
Jam without sugar added*
Raw local honey
Active Manuka honey
Organic Blackstrap Molasses

Herbs and Spices: Store in a cool and dry cabinet away from steam.
FYI- take the time to use fresh garlic and onion always!
Basil
Black Peppercorns and mill
Cardamom seed, ground
Cayenne pepper
Celery seed, ground
Celtic Sea Salt brand salt (not white salt)
Cinnamon, twig and ground
Coriander, ground
Cumin
Dill
Fennel Seed
Frontier Organic Adobo powder (Mexican)
Frontier Organic Chili powder (Southwest)
Frontier Organic Chinese Five Spice powder (Oriental)
Frontier Organic Curry powder (Indian, Thai)
Frontier Organic Herbs of Italy (Italian)

Frontier Organic Poultry Seasoning
Frontier Organic Pumpkin Pie Spice
Marjoram
Oregano
Sage
Tarragon
Thyme

<u>**Additional Dry Goods:**</u> store in a cool and dry cabinet away from
steam
Arrowroot
Baking powder (aluminum-free)
Baking soda
Sucanat
Decaffeinated coffee or Teechino
White Tea
Green Tea
Black Tea
All purpose flour (regular organic or gluten-free)
Buckwheat pancake/waffle mix (gluten-free is available)
Bread crumbs (gluten-free is available)
Blue cornmeal
Unbleached coffee filters
Unbleached parchment paper
Unbleached cheesecloth

<u>**Whole Grains:**</u> eventually you may get boxed mixes from the health
food store, first start with these basics
Steel-cut Oats or Gluten-free oats
Brown Basmati Rice
Long grain brown rice
Long grain wild rice blend

Quinoa and/or Quinoa instant flakes
Millet
Amaranth
Bob's Red Mill brand Meusli (this is not gluten-free)
Ancient Harvest brand Quinoa Polenta
Hodgeson Mill Whole Wheat or Gluten-free pasta brands mentioned earlier [limited amount, keep different styles on hand]
Alvarado Street Bread products
Ezekiel products- breads, granolas

Canned/Bottled Foods: these are intended for long term storage, basically the stuff you can stock up on, and can always use in a pinch when refrigerator is getting bare!
Wild Alaskan salmon
Chunk light tuna (limit)
Sardines[1]
Black beans
Kidney beans
Garbanzo beans
White beans
Black eyed peas
Eden Foods bean blends
Amy's brand Vegetarian Refried Beans
Amy's brand Vegetarian Baked Beans
Cascadian Farm brand Suerkraut
Cascadian Farm brand Pickles
Black Olives
Green Olives
Calamata Olives
Artichoke Hearts, preferably packed in water
Sundried Tomatoes in olive oil
Roasted Peppers in olive oil

What the Bleep $#@! Can I Eat?

Stuffed grape leave Dolmas
Sliced beets, if you can find them organic or just packed in water
Muir Glen Pizza Sauce
Muir Glen Fire Roasted Diced tomatoes (a must have!)
Muir Glen tomato products in general
Pasta sauce, tomato based
Just brand Pomegranate Juice
Just brand Purple Grape Juice
Just brand Black Cherry Juice
Knudsen Vegetable Juice

<u>Refrigerator Items:</u> in addition to the refrigerated condiments listed above
<u>Dark leafy cooking greens</u>- kale, chard, escarole, beet greens, turnip greens, broccoli raab
<u>Dark leafy salad greens</u>- spinach, arugala, mesclun mix, chickory, leaf lettuce, romaine
<u>Green foods</u>-asparagus, green beans, zucchini, broccoli, brussel sprouts, cucumber, peppers, celery, snow peas, kiwi, avocado
<u>Yellow-orange foods</u>-carrots, sweet potato, yams, peppers, tomatoes, beans, mango, papaya, lemons, onions, potatoes, yellow squash, cauliflower
<u>Red foods</u>- beets, tomatoes, strawberries, raspberries, radishes, peppers, pink grapefruit, red potatoes
<u>Purple foods</u>- artichoke, asparagus, eggplant, blueberries, blackberries, plums, figs, grapes, red onion
<u>Herbs</u>- scallions, parsley, cilantro, ginger root, and grow the rest
<u>Dairy-case Items</u>- organic Greek low-fat yogurt, organic low-fat ricotta, grated pecorino sheepmilk romano, whole milk fresh deli mozzarella balls (not pre-packaged), organic Fat-Free Milk [Lactose free available or goatmilk product substitutes if cow milk allergy], goat-sheep feta, cage free omega-3 eggs, tofu, tempeh

What the Bleep $#@! Can I Eat?

Freezer Items: keep it simple for now, prepared packaged food requires scrutiny for ingredients

Frozen Fish- [these are available at larger grocers and discount warehouses, these are also unflavored, vacuum packed, and possibly flash frozen] Wild Alaskan Sockeye Salmon, Wild caught Cod Fillets, Wild Alaskan Flounder Fillets, Wild caught Haddock, Wild caught Mahi Mahi, Wild caught Halibut

Frozen vegetables- green beans, corn, peas, asparagus, mixed vegetables (unseasoned), artichokes if you can find them frozen

Frozen Fruit- strawberries, blackberries, mixed berries, dark cherries

Bread Products- organic corn tortillas, Food for Life/Ezekiel products (not all gluten-free)

Meat Case: organic, free-range, hormone-free, low-fat, lean options

Poultry- Ground turkey 97-99% lean, Whole chicken (cut into 8 pieces or left whole), individually wrapped boneless skinless breasts, organic whole turkey when available, turkey tenderloin or breast

Beef- Organic or Natural Certified Angus London Broil, Stew Meat, Minute steaks, or ground buffalo

Lamb- Australian raised is my first choice, Loin chops, Rib chops, Leg of Lamb

Seafood- wild large sea scallops, wild sea bass, wild red snapper (my absolute favorite!), wild Alaskan salmon, halibut, haddock

Prepared Items- [LIMIT THE USE OF ALL OF THESE ITEMS!] Al Fresco sausages, Applegate Farm Items (turkey bacon, hot dogs, deli meat), some Boars Head products

RECOMMENDED COOKBOOKS/FOODBOOKS/MAGAZINES
The Rodale Whole Foods Cookbook
Gabriel Cousens, Conscious Eating and Spiritual Rainbow Diet
Paul Pitchford, Healing with Whole Foods
Sally Fallon & Mary G. Enig, Nourishing Traditions

John Robbins, Diet for A New World
Rombauer & Becker, Joy of Cooking (all the essentials)
Eating Well Magazine
Living Without Magazine and website
New England Naturopathic website- recipes and nutrition information
[www.drdebraanastasio.com, New England Naturopathic tab].

PREFERRED COOKING METHODS
Raw Whenever Possible/Appropriate- Basically all your fruits and salad vegetables can be eaten raw. Aim for 50-75% of your produce intake to be uncooked.
Daily produce intake recommendations:
- ½ cup berries
- 1 pom fruit- with seeds in the middle, plucked off a tree
- 1 stone fruit- with a pit in the middle, plucked off a tree
- 2 cups dark leafy greens
- 3-4 other ½ cup servings of vegetables (non-starchy preferably)
- Here's what doesn't count towards nutritional intake- processed fruit juice, jam, ketchup, French fries, potato chips, spinach tortillas, etc. Only real fruits and vegetables count towards healthy eating so focus on those.

If you can't imagine eating your daily requirements, then consider using a juice extractor and drinking it. Your only other option is dehydrated food powders at the health food store, but these are not nearly the same benefit as actually eating fruits and vegetables.
Raw seafood has advantages of the omega-3 content not being damaged, but there is a risk of gastrointestinal infection from bacteria or parasites. Sushi chefs are specially trained to select certain fish and prepare them to avoid infections. There is a good reason why wasabi and ginger slices are served with sushi, they kill germs and stimulate digestion! So don't skip the accompaniments, they are necessary.

Also, if you have good strong stomach acid and are not guzzling water at your meal, then most [but not all] germs from food are killed on contact (see chapter on Optimizing Digestion).

Steamed- A simple expandable metal steamer basket insert is a must have cooking item in the kitchen. I do not recommend microwave steaming due to the high core heat damaging the vitamins and protein of the food. The best vegetables for steaming are your broccoli family, string beans, greens, squashes, and potatoes as long as you only steam to the point where the vegetables retain brilliant color and are still a little crunchy. I also steam fish and sometimes chicken. The steamer basket is also great for reheating leftovers. I have been known to steam a late evening dinner.

Quick Steamed Dinner
3 oz. piece frozen fish, brussel sprouts cut in half, sweet potato cut into 1" cubes, steam for 20 minutes, add a drizzle of tamari and EVOO, done!

Sautéed- You don't always have to use oil for sautéing, consider the use of vegetable broth instead. Always keep the heat around medium without loud sizzling of the food. When you are sautéing, generally 1-2 T. of oil goes in the pan first, then the onion family items to season the oil, then the meat, then the rest of the vegetables (put the hardest ones in first, then the soft ones later). Most of the time you need to take the meat out of the pan to avoid scorching while the vegetables cook, so keep an eye on browning of your food items. The good part of sautéing is most everything is in one pan and it's relatively quick, the bad part is you absolutely have to stand with it and not leave it alone. Lastly, you can make your sauté with the same food items, and just by changing the seasoning you have a different meal [see the Frontier Organic spice blends in your pantry list].

THREE BASIC INGREDIENT DINNERS

- Chicken/Tofu- 3-4 oz. per person
- Onions & peppers- ¼ of each per person
- Baby Spinach- heaping handful per person

<u>Curry powder</u>, chick peas and coconut milk turn this into an Indian dish- serve over brown basmati rice (add a handful of cashews and currents to the rice while cooking)

<u>Chili powder</u>, black beans and lime juice turn this into a southwest dish- serve as fajitas in a whole grain wrap with Near East brand Spanish Rice Mix

<u>Chinese Five Spice powder</u>, mung bean sprouts and Tamari turns this into an Oriental dish- serve with broken Jasmine rice

<u>Herbs of Italy</u>, white beans, and diced tomatoes turns this into an Italian dish- serve with Lundberg brand Parmesan Risotto (this one you have to try!- just watch the sodium intake)

It's that easy to put together meals that contain vegetables and fiber without chemicals and gooey artificial thickeners. You can add more vegetables to get these meals even healthier. Believe me, these all taste great, the spices are high in antioxidants, the beans add fiber, and they are quick and easy to prepare. So, try each one to see what you like!

BAKED/GRILLED MEAT DINNERS

Baking heats up the kitchen and grilling takes the heat outdoors, but you can virtually do the same style of preparation whether you're in the kitchen or out on the grill. You will need a general cookbook to guide you for cooking a whole chicken, turkey or roast, or you can purchase the pop up timers and insert them as directed to guide your cooking. Basic prep of large cook items is as follows:

- <u>Whole chicken or turkey</u>- remove contents in cavity, rinse entire bird, pat dry, place in roaster pan breast side up. Rub entire bird with EVOO, sprinkle with Celtic Sea Salt and Poultry Seasoning (generously), water to cover bottom of pan, and stuff cavity with one medium onion cut into wedges, a chopped clove of garlic, and fresh herbs if you have them (rosemary, thyme, marjoram). Cover tips of wings with a little foil. Baked covered for initial 20 minutes, then uncover and baste every 15-20 minutes adding water to pan if needed until cooked to completion [follow cookbook instructions].
- <u>Lamb Roast</u>- rinse entire roast, pat dry, place in roaster pan with fat side up. Make slits in fat to insert cloves of garlic (many), pour dry vermouth over entire roast, sprinkle with Celtic Sea Salt, ground black pepper and thyme leaf (generously), follow cookbook instructions for cooking to completion.

Most everything else is cooked at 350 degrees for approximately 30 minutes depending on the thickness of the meat and whether or not the bone is in. Grilling is done on medium-high heat with the lid closed and no flashing/blackening of the meat.

- **Lamb loin steak, a bag of baby carrots, a bag of baby red/purple potatoes, and a handful of fresh herbs (thyme, rosemary, oregano)**- place in a glass pan, add Celtic sea salt, ground pepper and generous amount of thyme, put a little water in the bottom of the pan, cover with foil, bake, remove foil near the end of cooking time. For the grill, use a foil grilling bag or smoker bag with built-in wood chips, grill according to bag directions. Serve with greens and beans.

- **Halibut, acorn squash, asparagus and a handful of dillweed-** Place items in a glass baking dish as follows: halibut pieces in the center of the pan, wedges of acorn squash at ends of the pan, asparagus along the length of the pan, put slices of lemon and dill on top of the fish pieces, drizzle EVOO over the entire contents, put a little water in the bottom, cover with foil, bake, remove foil for 5-10 minutes before complete. On the grill, use a grilling basket, cut the acorn squash into ¼" rings, arrange items in basket, drizzle olive oil on everything, lemon juice on the fish, grill to completion without scorching. Add a drizzle of pure maple syrup and a sprinkle of cinnamon to the squash, and serve with brown rice.
- **Whole chicken cut into 8 pieces, sweet potato, zucchini-** rinse chicken pieces, pat dry, coat in olive oil and poultry seasoning and place into glass baking dish, cut potato into long Texas style fries and toss in olive oil, salt and pepper add to baking dish, cut zucchini into long strips and lay across the top of everything, water to cover bottom of pan, cover with foil for the first half of cooking, remove for the rest, cook to completion (30-40 minutes), serve with a wild rice blend.

DAILY MEAL PLANS- BASICALLY, WHAT TO EAT?

I know that adopting a healthy diet can make you feel lost. Think of this section as your tour guide to healthy eating. I would do it with you if I could, but now it's up to you. This takes a certain amount of courage, a sense of adventure, and a maturity to release any childish tendencies to just want goodies and junk. You are stepping into a way of life that is well suited for your entire mind and body. You are feeding your natural biochemistry and it is amazing what kind of changes you will experience. You will have your successes and your failures in the kitchen. You may initially be motivated to accomplish and then drift from your efforts seeking your old ways because this is the natural ebb and flow of making a change in your lifestyle. Be patient and kind to yourself in the process, don't judge it. Just keep trying to stay on track because in the end I know you will succeed in your quest for health by eating better!

BREAKFAST OPTIONS

The general construction of breakfast is to pick your protein first, sneak in vegetables whenever possible, eat berries, and add some whole grain, nuts, seeds or beans for fiber. Some options require very little prep, some are portable for commuting, and some are great for days when you have time to prepare a meal in the morning.

EGGS: cook them without browning or sizzling, use coconut oil in the pan, and limit an egg breakfast to only twice a week. Fast food egg breakfasts and most diners are not a suitable substitute because of the poor quality fats they are using, the use of high heat on the yolk, and the lack of any healthy items to go along with the egg.

- Poached/Over-Easy- place on a slice of Ezekiel toast, serve with strawberries and kiwi topped with a drizzle of coconut milk, macadamia nuts, ground chia seeds and grated ginger root.
- Soft/Hardboiled- eat 3 whites, 1 yolk, serve with steel-cut oats topped with walnuts, blueberries, ground flax seeds, drizzle of honey and cinnamon.
- Scrambled- whisk together 3 egg whites, 1 yolk and a little water, add vegetables that cook down easily (shredded zucchini or yellow squash, red pepper, tomatoes, spinach, leftover broccoli), serve with Food for Life English muffin
- Muffin Cup Crustless Quiches- see gluten free chapter for recipe, serve with a Lifestream Waffle
- Black Bean Breakfast Burrito- Ezekiel or Rice Tortilla, spread

with wholly guacamole, place scrambled egg (with spinach) in the middle, sprinkle on black beans, top with salsa and fold.

SOY: suited to those avoiding egg and/or dairy. Absolutely do not use processed soy! Only fermented soy in the form of tofu, tempeh, miso or tamari is beneficial. Limit to 4 full servings per week.

- <u>Scramble</u>- use soft tofu, mash with fork, lightly cook in pan with oil, add turmeric, Celtic sea salt and pepper. Serve with mixed berries topped a drizzle of coconut milk and sprinkle of granola.
- <u>Steak</u>- slice block of tofu or tempeh into ¼" thick rectangles, place in pan with raw onion slices, celtic sea salt and ground black pepper and lightly brown on one side, flip and add sliced raw mushrooms. Serve over baby spinach and with Ezekiel or Alvarado Street toast.
- <u>Smoothie</u>- 4 oz. soft tofu, ½ cup berries, 1 banana, 2 oz. coconut milk, 1 T. ground flax seeds, ½ cup pomegranate juice, and enough water for desired consistency while blending. Serve with one serving of any Ezekiel product. [Optional substitute: Jarrow Formulas Soy Essence is a fermented form of soy protein powder suitable for smooothies.]

<u>YOGURT:</u> organic, Greek is the preferred form because of the higher protein content, plain as opposed to pre-flavored, and low-fat or fat-free.

- <u>Parfait</u>- use a goblet or ice cream dish, layer in berries, Ezekiel or Udi's gluten-free granola, ground flax seeds and yogurt to provide a total of one serving of each item
- <u>Meusli</u>- yogurt mixed with Bob's Red Mill Meusli, let sit overnight in fridge or eat as is, add mixed berries, drizzle of honey, ground flax seeds, and a sprinkle of cinnamon

- Smoothie- 1 cup yogurt, ½ cup berries, ½ banana, 1 T. ground flax seeds, ½ cup Pomegranate juice, and water to desired consistency while blending. Be adventurous and add fresh mint or lemon balm to your smoothie! A serving of green powder supplement can also be added. Serve with one serving of an Ezekiel bread product.

POULTRY: especially well suited to those who wish to avoid dairy, egg and soy.

- Turkey Breakfast Patties- 1 lb. ground turkey, ground fennel seeds, Celtic sea salt, ground black pepper to taste formed into patties that fit intp the palm of your hand (3 oz.). Spread coconut oil on a cookie sheet, bake at 350 for 20-30 minutes, flip over halfway through. [serve one per person, freeze leftovers] Serve on top of baby spinach with blackberries on the side and a slice of Ezekiel or Alvarado Street toast . Tomato or vegetable juice goes fabulous with this, only a small amount though, 2-4 ounces.
- Turkey bacon- Applegate Farm Turkey Bacon, Food for Life waffle, real maple syrup, strawberries, 1 tsp ground flax seeds sprinkled on top with cinnamon.
- Chicken Breakfast Sausage- Al Fresco breakfast sausage, vegetable sauté of peppers, onions and spinach or breakfast hash if you have the time (recipe in the antioxidant chapter), served with Buckwheat pancakes (again if you have the time)/Lifestream waffle/Alvarado or Ezekiel toast.

BEEF: natural, certified angus or grass fed organic whenever possible. Use buffalo when available. These are sure to please the men of the house (I'm not being sexist, men need lots of zinc! So do growing children and pregnant women. Red meat is the highest food source of zinc, pumpkin seeds are the next best.) Limit to

just once or twice a week and one serving per person.

- Minute steaks- use coconut oil in the pan, place rings of raw onions and the steak in the pan, season with Celtic Sea Salt and ground black pepper, lightly brown on one side and flip, add mushrooms and simmer on low until cooked through. Serve over a handful of baby spinach with strawberries on the side and a slice of Ezekiel or Alvarado Street toast.
- Corned Beef- Boars Head corned beef, simmered with red cabbage and onions using water in the pan for the simmer, served with organic applesauce and dark cherries topped with ground flax seeds and cinnamon and a slice of whole grain toast. Goes well with English breakfast tea.
- Pastrami- Boars Head pastrami, sweet peppers in oil, sliced red onion, arugala and country style mustard on a whole grain English muffin or bread with mixed berries on the side.

LUNCH OPTIONS

Mid-day is a great time to get in a salad, some lean protein on the salad or in a sandwich, some beans, and raw vegetables in general. Simple dry crackers or flatbreads as a whole grain are well suited to this meal. Making an extra serving of protein at dinner the night before is especially helpful for quick lunch meal construction. Having batches of cold bean or grain salads is also a helpful addition to lunch.

- 1-2 cups of salad greens
- 2-3 servings of non-starchy vegetables, ½ cup each- cucumber, tomato, peppers, squashes, snow peas, green beans, radishes, artichokes, celery
- EVOO and lemon juice or apple cider vinegar (must include an acid on your greens, Celtic Sea Salt and ground pepper to taste. Dried or fresh herbs as desired. [optional dressings: Bragg Organic Healthy Vinaigrette or
- 3-4 oz. of lean protein- tofu, egg whites, chicken, fish, beef

- ½ cup beans- black, garbanzo, kidney, black-eyed peas, lentils
- 1 serving of a thin whole grain- WASA whole grain crackers, Mary' Gone Crackers, Ezekiel pita or tortilla

Lunch #1: Lentil soup, salad, turkey sandwich
Canned lentils, rinsed & drained, add to Pacific vegetable broth, add chopped parsley if desired. Greens and salad vegetables. Applegate Farm or Boars Head sliced turkey on whole grain pita with avocado or guacamole and shredded carrots.

Lunch #2: Black bean soup, salad, chicken fajita wrap
Black beans, rinsed and drained, added to Pacific vegetable broth, with a heaping tablespoon of salsa. Greens and salad vegetables. Ezekiel tortilla, 3 oz. chicken breast, avocado or guacamole, baby green and roll into a wrap.

Lunch #3: Turkey chili, salad, blue cornbread
1 cup Turkey chili recipe from the fiber chapter, greens and salad vegetables, recipe for cornbread on the package of blue cornmeal. My recommendation is to make these for a Sunday lunch so you can have leftovers for the next 1-2 days.

Lunch #4: Three Bean salad, chicken breast/tofu on salad, WASA crackers
Three bean salad recipe from fiber chapter, plain grilled chicken left over from dinner the night before or tofu cut into cubes, greens and salad vegetables and WASA crackers.

Lunch #5: Curried chicken/tofu, spinach salad, hummus w/crackers
Curried chicken/tofu recipe in the antioxidant chapter, spinach with tomatoes salad, 2 T. hummus on 1 serving of crackers.

Lunch #6: black bean chutney on tofu/fish, guacamole on crackers, salad. Black bean chutney recipe from fiber chapter on top of plain tofu or plain baked fish, 2 T. guacamole with crackers, greens and salad vegetables.

Lunch #7: Black Eyed Pea salad, hard boiled eggs on spinach salad
Black eyed pea recipe in the fiber chapter, 2 hard boiled eggs on spinach with mushrooms and red onions.

DINNER OPTIONS
The success of dinner depends on many factors such as time, number of people, taste preferences and how well a household is organized to have ingredients on hand for healthy meals. Out of all the meals, dinner can be the most intimidating for making changes in the diet. However, the most flavorful dinners can be achieved when cooking in the kitchen and this is your chance to prep for lunch for the next day.

Start by rotating the proteins you cook with, then rotate the styles of cooking by using spice blends. Some people never eat beans, fish or tofu and rely of just chicken and turkey. This type of eating is very limiting, especially nutritionally, so you have to be very creative to avoid tastebud boredom that makes you reach for more exciting things like manufactured salty and sugary foods.

If you already have recipes you like, amend them by taking away any bad fats, lower your cooking temps, steam or eat raw whatever you can, and add EVOO after cooking whenever possible.

Chicken Dinners:
- Baked chicken breast- glass dish, using the vinaigrette recipe

or Bragg Healthy vinaigrette drizzle over each peace, sprinkle with whole grain bread crumbs and a sprinkle of Herbs of Italy, Celtic sea salt and ground black pepper. Bake covered at 360 degrees for 30 minutes, remove foil for a few minutes at the end.

- Stir-fried chicken breast- use coconut oil, stir-fry on medium with onions, add vegetables such as red pepper, snow peas, green onions, bok choy, and mung beans, add Chinese Five Spice powder and tamari. Remove a large spoonful of juices from the pan and whisk together with 1 T. arrowroot starch, return the liquid to the pan and simmer until a glaze forms.
- Baked whole chicken/parts- see previous section on cooking a whole chicken, consult a cookbook on cooking chicken pieces with the bone in. Use EVOO and Poultry Seasoning.
- Braised Chicken pieces- dredge the chicken in seasoned flour, use coconut and EVOO in the pan to brown on each side, add vegetables and a flavored liquid such as vegetable broth or diced tomatoes and simmer.
- Chicken Kabobs- skewer chicken pieces and vegetables, use Antioxidant All-Purpose Marinade, lightly broil or grill turning every 10 minutes to avoid blackening.
- Chicken soup- the quick version of soup preparation is to sauté onions and garlic in EVOO at the bottom of a soup pot, add Pacific Chicken broth, pull the meat off of a whole cooked chicken breast, add a bag of Cascadian farms vegetable blend of peas/carrots/corn, add a handful of minced parsley, a generous sprinkle of herbs of Italy, and then my secret ingredients are a Tablespoon of honey, the juice of one fresh lemon and a sprinkle of ground cardamom.
- Chicken Chili- use leftover cooked chicken breasts cut into cubes, sauté a whole onion and a crushed clove of garlic in the bottom of the pot with EVOO, add white beans (rinsed,

drained), fresh cauliflower cut into 1" pieces, red potatoes with the peel cut into 1" cubes, Pacific vegetable broth, and chili powder, cook on low to keep bubbling until potatoes cooked through. Add a handful of chopped cooking greens near the end of cooking time.

- Chicken sausage & peppers- Using Al Fresco or Applegate chicken sausage cut into bit sized pieces, sauté onions, peppers and crushed garlic in EVOO, add the sausage and either diced tomatoes or pasta sauce.

Turkey Dinners:
- Baked whole turkey- see instructions above
- Baked turkey breast- you can find either with bone in or as a tenderloin, follow cooking instructions of package and season with EVOO and Poultry Seasoning
- Turkey meatballs- using the leanest natural turkey, mix in bowl with minced onion, crushed garlic, generous amount of dried or minced parsley, whole grain or gluten-free breadcrumb, and then I use whatever pasta sauce I have to make the ingredients come together to a consistency for forming 1" balls. Grease a cookie sheet with coconut oil, place balls on pan, use Misto to spray EVOO over all the meatballs, bake on top rack at 350 degrees until cooked through, turning them over after 15 minutes.
- Turkey burgers- you can use plain turkey meat or add your favorite natural seasonings. Either broil or grill to completion.
- Turkey Soup- using cooked turkey cut into bite sized pieces, sauté onion and crushed garlic in EVOO in the bottom of a soup pan, add Pacific chicken broth, slice carrots, minced parsley, and cut green beans. Add enough water to cover soup ingredients. In separate pan, cook wild rice, add cooked rice to the soup, add more water to the pan, add dried or fresh herbs

for seasoning.
- Turkey chili- see recipe in fiber chapter

Beef Dinners:
- Grilled London Broil- Using Antioxidant All-Purpose Marinade, Grill 10 minutes on one side, to completion on the second side, do not press on the meat to encourage flashing, only use enough marinade to avoid flaming, keep heat on medium with the lid closed and avoid blackening.
- Beef Stew- Using stew pot, sauté meat cut into small pieces and onion in EVOO in the pot, add one package of carrots sliced, one bag of baby gourmet potatoes, a pound of green beans, a handful of minced parsley, Pacific beef broth, Herbs of Italy, Celtic sea salt and ground black pepper to taste.
- Stir-fried beef- natural certified angus cut into strips, onions, peppers, mushrooms, green onions, baby bok choy, grated ginger, crushed clove of garlic, tamari, a drizzle of honey or maple syrup, crushed red pepper to taste.
- Buffalo Burgers- 3-4 oz. meat per burger, grill with All-purpose marinade. Serve with sliced red onion, sliced tomatoes, roasted red peppers, and leaf lettuce. Skip the cheese.

Lamb Dinners:
- Broiled Lamb Loin Chops- marinate chops in vermouth and a generous sprinkling of thyme for at least an hour, broil 10 minutes on one side, 5-7 minutes on the second side.
- Grilled Lamb Rib Chops- marinate in lemon juice, olive oil, crushed garlic and a generous sprinkling of oregano for at least an hour, grill 5-7 minutes on each side. Goes well with a wedge of iceburg lettuce, shredded red cabbage, sliced red onion, grape tomatoes and All Purpose Vinaigrette.
- Lamb and Lentil Stew- in a skillet, brown ground lamb with

minced onion, drain, add lentils to skillet (rinsed, drained), add a small can of diced tomatoes, season with Celtic Sea Salt, ground black pepper, oregano, marjoram, thyme.

Fish Dinners:

- Baked fish fillets- in glass baking dish, place fish fillets skin down, place a sliced onion and lemon on top of each fillet, drizzle all purpose vinaigrette over each fillet, sprinkle with whole grain breadcrumb (optional).
- Herb & Vegetable Stuffed Fish- see recipe in Omega chapter
- Fish Kabobs- cubed firm fish (salmon, bass, haddock, halibut), red pepper, onion, pineapple, dark cherries, all purpose marinade.
- Salmon burgers- preformed wild Alaskan salmon patties without additives such as breading/egg are available. Grill according to package instructions.
- Fish stew- white fish, scallops, clams, onion, potatoes, celery, vegetable broth, milk, parsley, Celtic sea salt, ground black pepper, corn kernals (fresh or frozen).

Tofu/Tempeh Dinners:

- Baked tofu/tempeh- place slices in glass baking dish, drizzle with EVOO and season to taste, bake at 350 for 20 minutes.
- Stir-fried tofu/tempeh- onions, peppers, bok choy, green onions, mushrooms, mung bean sprouts, tamari, Chinese Five Spice powder.
- Braised tofu/tempeh- dredge each piece in seasoned flour, using coconut and olive oil in skillet, lightly brown each side. Add vegetables such as mushrooms, chopped tomatoes, artichoke hearts and vegetable broth. Simmer to completion.
- Tofu kabobs- skewer cubes of tofu, zucchini, yellow squash, peppers and onions. Lightly grilled using all purpose marinade.

Bean Dinners

- <u>Vegetarian Chili</u>- in pot place chopped onion and peppers with EVOO in pan and lightly sauté, add beans of all kinds (rinsed, drained), add a large can of diced tomatoes, Chili powder, Celtic sea salt to taste. Serve over Yukon gold potatoes.
- <u>Beans and Rice</u>- Sauté onion and garlic with EVOO in pot, add dry rice, open large can of diced tomatoes and use the liquid toward the water portion to cook the rice. Near the end of the rice cooking time, add the diced tomatoes and black beans (rinsed, drained), Herbs of Italy, Celtic Sea Salt and ground black pepper to taste.
- <u>Bean burgers</u>- food process onions, peppers or zucchini for an amount to equal the amount of mashed black beans you have. Place together in a bowl, add some seasoned bread crumb and Amy's cream of mushroom soup to bring it together. Grill on foil or bake on tray to completion.
- <u>Bean Soup</u>- you can use Pacific broth and canned beans to quickly assemble a soup, or use the mixes from Bob's Red Mill which are wonderful and cook up beautifully in the crock pot.

SIDE DISHES

Greens- use a variety of greens for cooking, experiment with putting beans in the recipe, and change your spice choices to make each batch taste exciting and different.

- <u>Steam</u> in pot on stove until just wilted but still bright green, toss in EVOO, crushed garlic and lemon juice or apple cider vinegar.
- <u>Sauté</u> in skillet on medium heat with garlic, EVOO, and lemon juice.
- <u>Cook</u> Applegate turkey bacon and crumble, black eyed peas

(rinsed, drained), and onions all sauted in coconut oil, add greens and wilt them lightly, remove from heat, add Celtic Sea salt and ground black pepper. Add some spicy pepper flakes if desired.

Rice/grains- having a rice cooker is an enormous time saver. Cooking rice/grain in a pot is only as fast as the grain will allow, cooking it on high does not speed up the process and just evaporates the water you needed to complete cooking. Quick "Minute" mixes are discouraged since processing the grain takes away the nutritional benefits and are likely unhealthy in how they are processed and seasoned. You can use water, broths or the juice of diced tomatoes as the liquid portion of the grain cooking. For all grains, first bring the liquid portion to a boil, then add the grain, and lower heat to a soft simmer with the cover ajar to let out steam. Do not stir until the end of the cooking time using a fork to fluff the grain, adding any nuts, dried fruits, beans, or veggies that you desire.

1 cup grain	Liquid to cook	Time to simmer
Amaranth	3 cups	15 minutes
Quinoa	2 cups	15 minutes
Bulgur wheat	2 cups hot water	15 minutes, off heat
Millet	3 cups	25-30 minutes
Steel-cut oats	4 cups	20 minutes
White basmati rice	2 cups	20 minutes
Brown basmati rice	2 cups	30 minutes
Brown rice	2 cups	30-40 minutes
Wild rice blend	2 cups	50 minutes

Vegetables- include them whenever possible into the recipe of your main protein or grain. Most of all, get a variety of color and texture, and eat both raw and cooked.

- Steamed- never microwave, instead lightly steam using a

stovetop pan and steamer basket or a controlled temperature steamer without plastic pieces exposed to heat and food. It is best to attend to the pot to avoid overcooking, you want the vegetables brightly colored and still slightly crunchy.

- Prima Vera- almost anything can be served 'prima vera' meaning the season of Spring in Italian, using many vegetables and herbs together. Seafood, tofu, chicken or just a plan grain can be prepared in this manner.
- Tian- vegetables cut into thin pieces layered in a baking dish with something between them like cheese or egg creates a French inspired dish called Tian. I have done this on occasion when you have a little of each kind of vegetable left in the fridge and just want to use it up. Drizzle vegetables with olive oil every one to two layers in a shallow baking dish. Optional to top with seasoned bread crumb and or pecorino romano. Bake at 350 degrees until cooked together about 20 minutes.

SNACKS

A snack should serve the purpose of giving you energy, stabilizing blood sugar, and adding calories to the diet for those who need it. To serve this purpose, the snack should focus on protein, a little plant fat naturally in the food itself, and a fresh fruit or vegetable to go with it. Any added carbs should be in their whole grain (but not commercial products such as Triscuits or Wheat Thins, these are not healthy whole grains. Refer to your pantry shopping list for options. The best thing to do is examine your current snacking habits and try to decide what a suitable replacement is based on your taste preferences and then satisfy your taste buds using healthy, fresh foods. Shortcuts such as bars or drinks are not going to get you healthy because they are loaded with sugar and contribute to fatigue, weight gain, and blood sugar disorders.

- Hummus- organic, premade in many flavors, serve with fresh cut vegetables and whole grain crackers (optional).

- <u>Layered bean dip</u>- using a glass baking dish, place one can of Amy's Organic refried beans in a smooth layer at the bottom, cover with one package of Wholly guacamole in a smooth layer, cover with a generous amount of fresh salsa, top with shredded Mexican blend cheese (optional) and black olives (optional). Serve with fresh cut vegetables.
- <u>Artichoke dip</u>- one can artichokes packed in water, drained; one package Cascadian Farm spinach, thawed, drained; one can white beans, rinsed drained; 1-2 cloves garlic crushed; place ingredients in food processor and drizzle olive oil until a suitable paste consistency for dipping. Add Celtic Sea Salt and ground black pepper to taste. Serve with whole grain crackers and raw vegetable sticks.
- <u>Nut butters</u>- a serving of 1-2 Tablespoon with a cut up pear or apple is a suitable snack for mid-morning or mid-afternoon to bridge the gap between meals and avoid junk food or chocolate cravings.
- <u>Fruit & Protein</u>- a whole piece of fruit with the peel and a serving of yogurt, cottage cheese, ricotta, nuts or nut butter.
- <u>Meat & Vegetables</u>- sometimes it's nice to have 2-3 ounces of chicken, turkey or fish with some fresh cut vegetables dipped in All Purpose Vinaigrette to get through the afternoon.

RESTAURANT DINING TIPS

Learn to take your time when ordering out so that you can make the best choices possible for healthy eating. It is always best if you can view the menu prior to being seated, then there is no pressure to order if you can't find anything healthy on the menu. Remember you don't "deserve" the crummy food I have been telling you to avoid. Instead, you deserve to live a healthy life without disease or being dependent on toxic medications. I don't care what your taste buds want, they are part of the illness until you adopt a healthy eating plan. The taste buds will eventually come around to liking your new food choices.

SAMPLE MENU

Sun	Mon	Tues	Wed	Thurs	Fri	Sat
Boiled Eggs Oats, walnuts, blueberries, flax, honey, cinnamon	Yogurt Parfait Toast	Turkey pattie Spinach Blackberries Toast	Tofu scramble Mixed berries, coconut milk, granola	Chicken Breakfast Sausage Onions, peppers, spinach Waffle	Smoothie	Steak w/ mushrooms Spinach Strawberries Toast
Apple, almonds	Pear, cashew	Grapes, sunflower seeds	Peach, Pecans	Plum, walnuts	Apricots, pistachios	Cherries, Almonds
Grilled London Broil Green beans Yellow squash Salad	LO Turkey chili Salad	LO Chicken as curry salad Green Salad Crackers	Salmon salad Salad Lentil Soup	Tofu Black Bean chutney Salad	Black eyed Peas and Eggs Salad	Fish Salad Crackers Salad
Turkey chili Potato Greens	Baked chicken Wild Rice Broccoli	Salmon Basmati rice Greens	Beans and rice Greens with garlic	Lamb Rice Pilaf Spinach	White fish Brown rice Greens	Kabobs Tabouli Cauliflower

TEN STEPS TO SUCCESSFUL DINING OUT

1. Look for any beans on the menu- peruse the appetizer section and main entrée descriptions. Order the beans as a side dish or on top of your salad.
2. Look for any artichokes on the menu- listed in the main entrée descriptions. Have these added to your main protein, on top of a salad, or as a side dish.
3. Look for any salmon, sea scallops, sea bass, halibut, haddock

on the menu and be ready to order it "baked or grilled with olive oil and lemon juice and no seasoning please."

4. Look for any greens such as kale, escarole or broccoli raab on the menu and have them prepared "without butter but instead with olive oil and garlic and no seasoning please."
5. Ask the wait staff to list all of the vegetables that are available as side dishes "without butter or seasoning please."
6. Then, take your chances and look for a whole grain, but the best it's going to get is whole grain bread or maybe some oatmeal. If you are traveling for more than a day, then take advantage of these grain options to avoid constipation. Otherwise just skip it for now until your next meal at home.
7. Instruct your wait staff to hold the bread but to "please bring olive oil, vinegar and lemon wedges to the table."
8. Remember to refuse the gigantic glass of water served with the meal. You can order a small bottle of sparkling mineral water and a few glasses to split it without ice and some lemon if you need a few sips with the meal.
9. Completely avoid the sweet drinks and the dessert menu. Sometimes there are real fresh fruit smoothies available that you can split and have as a dessert, but drinking your fruit is not as beneficial as eating your fruit .
10. If there is the outside chance of fresh fruit and nuts being available, have them served at the end of the meal to have with some organic tea. If you prefer, put the tea over ice and sip.

FOUNDATION NUTRITION SUPPLEMENTS

We have used many different brands of vitamins over the years and have abandoned one after the other for complaints of nausea and stomach upset. Now that we have our own vitamin line, we can provide a high quality multivitamin that is digestible.

- *Metamorphosis Products Foundation Multivitamin*™- (adult

and pediatric) provides a full array of vitamins and minerals in their most digestible and absorbable form with a suitable amount of Iron when needed for women and children.
- *Metamorphosis Products Calcium Essential™*- (capsule and chewable)-provides the correct forms of calcium and vitamin D for proper use in the body to correct and prevent bone and teeth disease.

WHERE DO YOU GO FROM HERE?
- After you have adopted your healthy diet for a minimum of three months, go and have your lipid panel and glucose markers checked to begin to see the fruits of your efforts.
- Make healthy food for family and friends when they visit you or you visit them. Remember they need to eat healthy too whether they are ill or not.
- Adopt a healthy outdoor life of walking, biking, swimming, tennis, gardening, journaling or photography for exposure to the benefits of nature.
- Help the children in your life by avoiding the junk snack food they are accustomed to and providing only healthy foods in your presence.
- When you are healthy and strong in your will, have only an occasional treat, but don't feel like you need to go back. It's always better to just look forward.
- Enjoy this process! You have invested not only in your own health, but in the many lives you touch with your presence. You will be missed if you leave this world prematurely, so keep yourself healthy so you can live a long and happy life!

"I am reminding myself of this as well. We are all on this journey together. God bless all of you!"—Dr. A

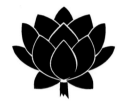

Chapter 10:
Treats & Cheats

As I type this, I wonder if you read the previous chapters or if you're jumping ahead. Hmmmm. Treats and Cheats are reserved for occasional use, during times of personal overload or crisis, or sometimes while traveling. Everyone wants shortcuts, but shortcuts are just that, they cut you short on something, namely nutrition. So as you read, please understand you are not getting proper nutrition from these options, but they are better than typical fast food, diners or other commercial foods that people typically turn to. Remember, it's what you do consistently that you either benefit or suffer from.

Breakfast Treats & Cheats:
Starbucks Turkey Bacon Eggwhite Breakfast Sandwich
Starbucks Oatmeal cup with toppings
Amy's Organic Black Bean Breakfast Burrito
Kashi Veggie Medley Pocket Sandwich
Odwalla Protein Smoothie
Bolthouse Farms Protein Smoothie
McDonalds Fruit & Yogurt Parfait

What the Bleep $#@! Can I Eat?

Snack Treats & Cheats:
Kashi TLC Bars
Cliff Z-Bars
Odwalla Bars
Omega smart nutrition bar
PureFit nutrition bar

Lunch/Dinner Treats & Cheats:
Kashi Frozen Meals, Frozen Pockets, Frozen Pizzas
Amy's Organic Meals, Organic Burritos, Organic Pizzas
Organic Bistro Frozen Meals
Cedarlane Organic Frozen Meals
Whole Foods 365 Frozen Meals

Beverage Treats & Cheats:
Zevia Natural Diet Soda
Virgil's Root Beer
Izze Sparkling Juice
Blue Sky Organic Soda
Jones Organic Iced Teas
Sweet Leaf Iced Teas
Polar Seltzer
Metromint Waters
Crop Organic Vodka
Organic Wine
Organic Microbrew Beer

Dessert Treats & Cheats:
Organic Nectars Raw Agave Gelato
Papalani Sorbetto & Gelato
Santa Cruz Organic Dessert Toppings- fruit and chocolate syrup

Natural Choice Sorbet and Fruit Bars
Purely Decadent Coconut Ice Cream
Alden's Organic Ice Cream
Organic Dark Chocolate- Newmans, Green & Black, Dagoba
Cookies-Barbara's Organics, Newmans Own

Now some of these are not at your regular grocer, but they are worth the trip to the health food store. Use them in small amounts, and only on occasion. These foods are to be savored, not devoured by the carton. Eventually you will learn how to do without these foods and use just real food instead. Create your own frozen dinners with food that you prepared. Stock up on a variety of food storage containers so you can freeze any leftovers for another day. And lastly, plan ahead so you don't need these shortcuts at all!

ENDNOTES

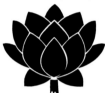

Introduction
[i] www.usda.gov, Dietary Guidelines for Americans, 2010.

Optimizing Digestion

[ii] Am J Clin Nutr. 2001 Feb;73(2 Suppl):444S-450S.Probiotics: effects on immunity.Isolauri E, Sütas Y, Kankaanpää P, Arvilommi H, Salminen S.Department of Pediatrics, the University of Turku, Turku, Finland. erika.isolauri@utu.fi

Optimizing Food Quality
[iii] www.ota.com Organic Trade Association
[iv] www.ehp.niehs.nih.gov/docs/2002/110-5/ss.html#harm Harmful Farming
[v] Ibid.
[vi] http://www.albany.edu/ihe/salmonstudy/pressrelease.html
[vii] www.usatoday.com/news/nation/2007-04-16-imported-food_N.htm Imported Food Rarely Inspected.
[viii] http://chemicallypure.com/barcodes-country-of-origin
[ix] Blaylock, Russel. 1997. Excitotoxins: The Taste that Kills. Health Press, Santa Fe, NM
[x] www.feingold.org
[xi] www.truthinlabeling.org, "There Are No Regulations for Labeling Processed Free Glutamic Acid (MSG).
[xii] www.cspinet.org, "Consumer Group Calls for Ban on "Flour Improver." Potassium Bromate Termed a Cancer Threat." July 19, 1999.
[xiii] US Food and Drug Administration: Center for Food Safety and Applied Nutrition "Questions and Answers on the Occurrence of Benzene in Soft Drinks and Other Beverages"

[xiv] www.fiengold.org "Many Learning and Behavior Problems Begin in Your Grocery Cart." 3/4/10

[xv] www.fiengold.org

[xvi] www.independent.co.uk "Caution: Some soft drinks may seriously harm your health. Experts link additive to cell damage." Martin Hickman, May 27, 2007.

[xvii] http://www.health.state.ny.us/environmental/lead/sources.htm

xviii Chemical BPA Used In Most Food Can Linings Raises Concerns, By Ernest Scheyder, June 10, 2010, www.insurancejournal.com/news/national/2010/06/10/110610.htm#ixzz0s8Xglah3

[xix] Alternatives to BPA containers not easy for U.S. foodmakers to find. By Lyndsey Layton,Washington Post Staff Writer ,Tuesday, February 23, 2010

[xx] http://www.aboutgoatmilk.info/goat-milk/goat-milk-is-more-beneficial-to-health-then-cow-milk/

[xxi] http://www.edenfoods.com/articles/view.php?articles_id=80

Low Glycemic Diet

[xxii] www.ncbi.nlm.nih.gov/pubmed/400272 Acta Vitaminol Enzymol. 1979;1(1-6):5-10. [Vitamin C and phagocytic system: present status and perspectives (author's transl)] [Article in Italian] Patrone F, Dallegri F.

[xxiii] Journal of Orthomolecular Medicine, 1999; Vol 14 (3): 143-56. Ascorbic Acid and Some Other Modern Analogs of the Germ Theory John T. A. Ely, Ph.D.Radiation Studies, Box 351310
University of Washington Seattle, WA 98195

xxiv www.jimmunol.org/cgi/content/abstract/89/3/314 The Journal of Immunology, 1962, 89, 314 -317 Copyright © 1962 by The American Association of Immunologists, Inc. The Effects of Alloxan Diabetes on Phagocytosis and Susceptibility to Infection Kenneth F. Wertman and Mary R. Henney

[xxv] www.laleva.cc/food/aspartame_factsheet.htmlTHE BITTER TRUTH ABOUT ASPARTAME AND NEOTAME "Aspartame/Neotame - the most dangerous substances in our food supply today." - Mary Nash Stoddard [Founder ACSN & Pilot Hotline]

[xxvi] www.sparkaonline.com

[xxvii] www.splendaexposed.com New Splenda, Sucralose Study Reveals Shocking Potential Harmful Effects,Source: Chairman of Citizens for Health Declares FDA Should Review Approval of SplendaChairman of Citizens for Health Declares FDA Should Review Approval of SplendaNew Study of Splenda and Sucralose Reveals Shocking New Information About Potential Harmful Effect on Humans

xxviii www.ynhh.org/online/nutrition/advisor/sugar_alcohol.html

[xxix] http://www.living-foods.com/articles/agave.html

[xxx] Fructose. http://www.vitamins-supplements.org/carbohydrates/fructose.php

Antioxidant-Rich Diet

[xxxi] Oxygen Radical Absorbance Capacity (ORAC) of Selected Foods – 2007, Nutrient Data Laboratory, Beltsville Human Nutrition Research Center (BHNRC),

What the Bleep $#@! Can I Eat?

Agricultural Research Service (ARS), U.S. Department of Agriculture (USDA), Arkansas Children's Nutrition Center, ARS, USDA, Little Rock, AR, November 2007.
U.S. Department of Agriculture, Agricultural Research Service
Beltsville Human Nutrition Research Center, Nutrient Data Laboratory, 10300 Baltimore Avenue
Building 005, Room 107, BARC-West, Beltsville, Maryland 20705, Tel. 301-504-0630, FAX: 301-504-0632, E-Mail: ndlinfo@ars.usda.gov, Web site: http://www.ars.usda.gov/nutrientdata
[xxxii] Nashville, USA, in 2006 titled "Chlorogenic Acids and Lactones in Regular and Water Decaffeinated Arabica Coffee," (published in The Journal of Agriculture and Food Chemistry in 2001)
[xxxiii] "Comparison of the Antioxidant Activity of Commonly Consumed Polyphonic Beverages (Coffee, Cocoa, and Tea) Prepared per Cup Serving," which was published in The Journal of Agriculture and Food Chemistry in 2001
xxxiv http://www.sciencedaily.com/releases/2003/11/031106051159.htm Hot Cocoa Tops Red Wine And Tea In Antioxidants; May Be Healthier Choice ScienceDaily (Nov. 6, 2003)
xxxv www.mayoclinic.com Red Wine and Resveratrol: Good for your heart?

Omega 3 Balanced Diet

[xxxvi] http://www.nlm.nih.gov/medlineplus/druginfo/natural/patient-fishoil.html
[xxxvii] www.nutritiondata.com
[xxxviii] He K, Lio K, Daviglus ML et al. Intakes of long-chain n-3 polyunsaturated fatty acids and fish in relation to measurements of subclinical atherosclerosis. Am J Clin Nutr 2008 Vol. 88(4):1111-1118.

xxxix
Carcinogenesis, June 2010,Dietary olive oil and corn oil differentially affect experimental breast cancer through distinct modulation of the p21Ras signaling and the proliferation–apoptosis balance

[xl] BMC Cancer, 2009 Jan 30;9:42.Coherent anti-Stokes Raman scattering imaging of lipids in cancer metastasis.Le TT, Huff TB, Cheng JX. Weldon School of Biomedical Engineering, Purdue University, West Lafayette, IN 47907, USA. thuc@purdue.edu

xli Aguilera CM, Ramirez-Tortosa MC, Mesa MD, Gil A. [Protective effect of monounsaturated and polyunsaturated fatty acids on the development of cardiovascular disease]. Nutr Hosp 2001 May-2001 Jun 30;16(3):78-91 2001. PMID:11620.
[xlii] Virgin Olive Oil Linked to Protection Against Breast Cancer by a Number of Mechanisms, 01/01/2010. http://www.ecancermedicalscience.com/news-insider-news.asp?itemId=1102
[xliii] Diet and Fitness Today, Foods High in Fatty Acids, Total Monounsaturated.
[xliv] Benzene, Production, Import/Export, Use & Dispoal.http://www.atsdr.cdc.gov/toxprofiles/tp3-c5.pdf

[xlv] Fuhr U, Boettcher MI, Kinzig-Schippers M, et al. Toxicokinetics of acrylamide in humans after ingestion of a defined dose in a test meal to improve risk assessment for acrylamide carcinogenicity. Cancer Epidemiology Biomarkers and Prevention 2006; 15(2):266–271.

[xlvi] Lipids. 1998 Aug;33(8):821-3. Lectin may contribute to the atherogenicity of peanut oil. Kritchevsky D, Tepper SA, Klurfeld DM.The Wistar Institute, Philadelphia, Pennsylvania 19104, USA. kritchevsky@wista.wistar.upenn.edu

[xlvii] http://www.mayoclinic.com/health/trans-fat/CL00032
[xlviii] Facts on Olestra, Center for Science in the Pulbic Interest, http://www.cspinet.org/olestra/11cons.html
[xlix] Mary G. Enig, Ph.D., Director Nutritional Sciences Division Enig Associates, Inc.
[l] The Health Benefits of Eating Sardines. http://www.associatedcontent.com/article/497497/the_health_benefits_of_eating_sardines.html?cat=5